From the Seeds of Sadness

From the Seeds of Sadness

A MEMOIR

Gemma M. Geisman

Library of Congress Control Number: 2009903266
ISBN: Hardcover   978-1-4415-2612-0
                 Softcover   978-1-4415-2611-3

To order additional copies of this book, contact:
Xlibris Corporation
1-888-795-4274
www.Xlibris.com
Orders@Xlibris.com
59098

For my husband, Dick, who loved and supported
me throughout the entire journey.

For our children, Cathy, Mike, Cindy and Rick
who taught us so much about
unconditional love.

Prologue

Pain of heart and pain of soul are agonies that have been with us since the beginning of time. No human is immune. None can escape them. To me, though, it seems that the agony parents suffer for their incurably ill child is the most tormenting and devastating ache of all.

What I didn't know when our second child, Mike, was born with osteogenesis imperfecta (OI), a rare genetic defect, is how damaging the blunt realities of an incurable illness can be on the caregivers.

Truth about a disability is often difficult to swallow; it's so much easier to think in terms of hope. So instead of facing the realities of osteogenesis imperfecta, I buried them while I prayed for miracles and tried desperately to make our lives appear normal.

Bringing Mike home from the hospital instead of placing him in an institution, picking him up when I'd been told not to, and concentrating on his bright blue eyes and happy smile were positive ways of coping had they allowed the hidden, festering feelings to surface. But they didn't.

The words osteogenesis imperfecta were foreign and strange sounding to me, and no matter where I looked, or to whom I turned to for definitions and explanations, the refrain was always the same. "We're sorry. There is nothing else we can tell you. We're sorry. There is no cure. We're sorry. We're sorry. We're sorry." As a result, I shut out the words so obviously disconnected from hope and began living life in my own prison of impossible dreams.

Only God could deliver me from this self-imposed prison, and mercifully, he did. For one short perilous moment, life hung precariously in the balance. And it was only through his intercession that I was made to see what the power of love can do.

Because of this fateful discovery, I decided early in 1967 to write about my feelings about OI, my eventual acceptance of Mike's illness, and the gift of love that resulted. Then I sent it to *Redbook* magazine's Young Mother's Story series. I didn't really know why I did it. Writing it was a form of therapy, ridding me of so many mixed feelings and so much pain. It was like getting over a long, critical illness that had been too serious to discuss but could be talked about now that the crisis was over. Though a part of me didn't want to divulge my painful, personal journey, another part urged me to speak up. So it was with a bit of ambivalence that I deposited my manuscript in the mailbox.

Several months passed, and occasionally, I'd think about the article and wished that I had never sent it. To make myself feel better, I imagined it buried deep in a slush pile on some editor's desk. Or better yet, thrown into a wastebasket.

One day, after I had almost succeeded convincing myself that the article was gone for good, an envelope, appearing too thin to hold a returned manuscript and bearing a *Redbook* return address, was delivered. Uncharacteristic of a freelance writer, I ripped the envelope open hoping to find a standard rejection form. Instead, in it was a brief letter that read as follows:

Dear Mrs. Geisman:

Thank you for sending "My Prison of Dreams" to our Young Mother's Story series. We all found it very moving and compellingly honest and would like to publish it in our series. Before we reach a final decision, however, we would like to know if you are willing to have your story published with your name, the name of your town, and a picture, as is our custom. We ask you only because there is no covering letter from you saying one way or the other.

I read the letter over and over again, and still I couldn't believe that they wanted to publish my story. I really hadn't written it for publication but, rather, to renew myself so that I could start over again and be the kind of mother Mike deserved. I scolded myself for sending it instead of relegating it to a desk drawer; then I reminded myself that the choice was still mine. I could reject the magazine offer, put a halt to it right now. Ridden with indecision, I searched my heart for the right answer. I hadn't even told my husband, Dick, that I'd written a story about my feelings and sent it off to a magazine. What would he think when he found out?

That evening, after our four children were in bed, I handed him the *Redbook* letter without explanation. Puzzled, he read it. Finally, he put the letter down and asked, "Do you have a copy of the article?" I nodded and reluctantly handed him the copy I held behind my back.

As he read, I watched Dick's face go through a wide range of emotions that included pain, disbelief, sorrow, and finally, tender and understanding love.

"Why didn't you tell me you felt that way too?" he murmured softly.

Aghast, I looked into his pain-filled eyes. "You mean you too?"

"Yes," he admitted gruffly, "it's true, but I thought I could never tell you. You were always so upbeat, so positive. I never dreamed you were suffering so much inside."

I could hardly believe what I was hearing. All these long, terrifying years, we had never once shared our deepest thoughts about Mike's illness because we both had feared that it was shameful to have feelings we didn't understand. Now it was as if a floodgate had been opened, letting all the pent-up words pour out. That night, we talked for hours about everything that mattered, and afterward, Dick said, "Just look what your article has done for us. Say yes to *Redbook*. Maybe it will help other parents like us."

I hesitated. Telling a husband who loved me and telling the world were two different matters. Maybe the world wouldn't be as kind and understanding. "How can I bare my soul for all to see? What will our families think? What about our friends and neighbors?"

"They'll understand and love you all the more," he said. "And if some don't understand, we won't let them matter."

What people would think of me bothered me a great deal, but not as much as the thought that I might be exposing Mike to more pain and suffering by allowing my story about my ambivalent feelings to be published. I never doubted for a moment that my article stressed the gift of love, but would *he* understand that? After all, he was only a child. At eleven, he knew only too well about the pain of fractures, the cumbersomeness of plaster casts, and the limitations of a wheelchair. But was he mature enough to understand the emotional ramifications?

Talking to Mike about so grown-up a subject would be difficult, but I felt that it was important that I do so before making a final decision about publication. The next day, when Dick was at work and the other children in school, I approached him, put my arms around him, and hugged him tenderly. "Mom, stop it! You're going to break my arms," he laughed.

Without further preliminaries, I asked, "Mike, you know I love you, don't you?"

Grinning with embarrassment, he replied, "Sure, I do."

"I love you," I repeated, "but I *hate* osteogenesis imperfecta and what it's doing to you."

"I hate it too!" he said with such force, it surprised us both.

"Wow!" I said. "I'm glad that's out."

He sighed and leaned back in his wheelchair. "Yeah, me too."

"I wrote a story about how much I hated OI and what it was doing to you and me. And about how my feelings were so mixed up for a while, I didn't even know how I felt about you. *Redbook* magazine wants to publish that story."

He turned his eyes away, and almost timidly, he asked, "Did you hate me?" And before I could answer, he quickly added, "I wouldn't blame you if you did."

"I loved you from the first moment I saw you. I swear it from the bottom of my heart," I said, making the sign on my breast to seal the oath.

"Then there's no problem," he said with an even wider grin than before.

I picked the article up from a nearby table and asked, "Do you want to read it?"

"Naw," he said, waving me away, "whatever you said in it is okay with me."

Later, I spoke to Cathy, Cindy, and Dickie about the article. Seven-year-old Dickie wasn't at all concerned about it one way or the other, and the girls were simply impressed with the fact that their mom was going to be published in a national magazine.

With these hurdles cleared, Dick and I debated the issue of getting published anonymously or with my full name and the name of our town. Publishing anonymously would be much easier, I argued, but wouldn't that be the same as hiding from the very same problems we were trying to overcome, especially the problems we had encountered because of our buried, festering feelings? Wouldn't we be hiding away from the prospect of undeserved shame and fear, the way earlier generations of parents had hidden their handicapped children in closets or attics?

Dick agreed, and so the decision was made to allow *Redbook* to publish our story with my byline, a photo of our children, and any additional information they needed. I felt happy and relieved about our decision, yet I awaited publication for an entire year with a mixture of hope and fear. Little did I realize that once the article was published, our lives would never be the same again.

Part One

Chapter One

More than anything, we wanted a boy. My husband, Dick, had just been discharged from the navy. Having returned to his Ohio hometown, we were looking forward to moving into the small, cozy house that we'd rented, painted, and furnished with all-new furniture and appliances. It was to be our first real home after living in navy housing, and we could hardly wait to move in with the new baby and two-year-old Cathy.

Dick had just started a job, and so, because we would need someone to care for Cathy while I was in the hospital, we had opted to stay with his parents until after the birth, when the four of us would move into the house and begin our new lives.

Ultrasound wasn't available in the midfifties to predict the sex of our expected baby, but we just knew it would be a boy. Cathy's little pink nighties had been relegated to storage boxes, replaced by blue sleepers; and my sports-minded husband had bought an assortment of balls, a tiny baseball bat and glove, and other boy things.

Filled with many happy thoughts of dreams come true, I woke up during the early-morning hours on April Fool's Day and told Dick that the time had come to go to the hospital. We rushed there only to have the contractions fade, then intensify, fade, then intensify again. After I'd been there for hours, Dr. Burnes, a tall thin doctor with a wide smile and crew cut hair, told us he wanted to take x-rays to see if a problem existed. When he returned to the labor room minutes later, he seemed thoughtful and restrained. "What you're having is false labor," he said. "I'm going to send you home. When the contractions start up again, wait until they're strong and about five minutes apart, then call me."

Feeling somewhat embarrassed about going home without a baby, we tried to make light of it by passing it off as an April fool's joke.

During the week that followed, I continued to have contractions sporadically, and the same puzzling thing that had happened before happened again. I'd reported it to Dr. Burnes the first time, but he had only laughed and said I was imagining things. When I saw him the week after the false labor, I told him, "The other day, I crossed my legs and heard that cracking noise again."

This time, the young doctor didn't laugh. Still, he wouldn't speculate about the sound I'd heard. Instead, he gently patted me on the back and said something about hoping that I'd have the baby real soon.

By then, I was getting worried, but didn't want to voice it out loud to anyone. I desperately wanted the baby to be born soon and without complications. Yet when I again went into labor after midnight, the morning of Friday the thirteenth, I prayed that the contractions would stop like they had before. I didn't want our happily anticipated child to be born on a day cloaked with superstition and fear. But nothing, not even prayer, could stop the contractions that pushed Mike into the world at 3:43 a.m. on Friday, April 13.

Having experienced the cheerfulness of a maternity ward after Cathy's birth, I realized almost immediately that something was terribly wrong with the atmosphere that now surrounded me. Somber faces, clamped lips, and averted eyes would best describe what I saw.

A young blonde nurse padded around my bed, doing her duties quickly, acting oddly as if I had just come down with a contagious disease instead of giving birth to a baby. I felt oddly deflated—empty. My baby had been born. I vividly remembered the doctor and nurses exclaiming that I'd had a boy. And I remembered thinking how happy Dick would be before I'd given in to heavily induced sleep. So why was everyone acting as if I had the plague?

"Where's *my* baby?" I asked the nurse after cartfuls of babies had been delivered to every mother but me.

Looking confused, she said, "I can't bring him in right now. Dr. Burnes is still examining him."

Then she turned and almost ran out of the room.

I lay there alone, wondering where Dick was, thinking about the hubbub of the time when Cathy was born, about his gift of red roses, his kisses of congratulations, and the baby warm and new in my arms.

Several eternities seemed to pass before Dr. Burnes came in wearing the same guarded mask the others wore. Putting a large book aside on the bed stand, he pulled a chair close to my bedside and reached for my hand. *My god*, I thought, horrified. *He looks like the pitying, sympathizing faces at Papa's funeral!* I tried to smile, but suddenly, it hurt too much to even try.

"I have to talk to you about your baby," he said.

I told myself not to listen. I turned my head toward the wall and withdrew my limp hand from his. But no matter how hard I tried, I couldn't shut out his words.

"Gemma, you have a son," he said.

I turned and looked at him, not understanding. I had been so sure he was about to tell me my baby was dead. If he wasn't dead, then what?

"He was born with what we think is a rare, crippling bone disease called osteogenesis imperfecta," he said, enunciating the strange-sounding words. Then, his voice cracking, he continued, "We couldn't count them all on the x-rays, but we think he was born with somewhere between thirty to fifty fractures. Some of them occurred before he was born and have already healed."

"The cracking noise," I murmured while tears brimmed in my eyes at the thought of my baby breaking while I'd thought him safe in my womb.

"Probably," he said, averting my eyes. "But our concerns now are the fractures he suffered during delivery. His breech birth caused a lot of damage to his legs, as well as his arms, collar bones, and ribs."

"Did you know about this when you took x-rays during my false labor?"

Avoiding my question, he went on with explanations. "When the nurse was washing and dressing your baby, she noticed that one leg seemed rather limp. Thinking it could have fractured during the breech delivery, we x-rayed it. That's when we discovered both the old and new fractures and ordered full-body x-rays. I conferred, by phone, with several orthopedic specialists at a Fort Wayne, Indiana, hospital. They believe he may have osteogenesis imperfecta. They tell me that it's very rare and that there is no known cause or cure. Because he has so many fractures, they fear he may not live. For now, all they can do is cast the fractures and make him comfortable." Reaching for the book on the nightstand, he added, "I've never seen a case of osteogenesis imperfecta, nor do I know much about it other than what I could find in this textbook. Do you want me to read it to you?"

I didn't really want to hear it, but I nodded yes as hot tears filled my eyes and streamed down my cheeks. I was only twenty-one and knew little about medical terminology, so the detailed medical explanations made little sense to me.

And the symptoms—blue coloration of the sclera (a coating that covers part of the eyeball), the head malformation, the deformed limbs, along with the prognosis of frequent fractures and stunted growth to be expected if he survived—only served to frighten me more. Even the doctor seemed dazed by his own recitation. Putting the book down, he exclaimed, "There's no way you can take care of this baby at home. If he lives, I promise to do all I can to help you find an institution that will take him."

I felt hysteria mounting. I wanted my baby, and my husband. Oh my god! Where was Dick? How he must be hurting! "Where's Dick? Does he know?" I murmured.

"We phoned him at work. He came quickly, and we gave him a brief explanation, not all the details like I've just given you. He's on his way to Fort Wayne now with the baby. We thought it best to have him taken there so he could get the specialized care he needs."

"But I haven't even seen him yet," I sobbed.

He sighed. "I know. But we felt it was an emergency situation."

Stunned, I asked, "Dick went with him in the ambulance?"

"No, he's taking him by car."

"You mean you let him drive to Fort Wayne alone with a sick, maybe a dying baby?"

"I believe his mother went with him," he responded; then with another pat of the hand, he said, "I'll leave the book with you in case you want to read it again later on. I know it's too much for you to absorb right now." Then he was gone, leaving me to thrash out the nightmare alone.

They brought me food that I couldn't eat and medication to dull the pain, but I wouldn't take it. I wanted to be fully awake when Dick returned from his emergency trip to Fort Wayne.

When finally he arrived, later in the day, he rushed to my bedside and embraced me tenderly while his mother hung back in the shadows.

Feeling transfused by his strength, I found the courage to ask, "How's our little boy?"

"He's cute. He looks like me," he said with a smile. "Blond hair and big blue eyes."

"But how is he?" I repeated.

"He seemed okay. When Mom and I arrived at the emergency entrance of the hospital in Fort Wayne, a bunch of doctors and nurses were waiting for us. They took him right away and disappeared. I was asked to fill out some papers; then I was told that they would contact us as soon as they had fully evaluated his condition. All I know is that he had a broken leg, maybe a few other breaks, because he was born breech."

My heart sank. Was that all he had been told?

"You and Mom just left then, without seeing him again, without being told more than that?"

"Should we have stayed?" he asked, perplexed. "They told us to go, and I was anxious to get back to be with you." Searching my tearstained face, I think he realized then, for the first time, the true extent of the emergency. "It's more than just a few broken bones, isn't it?" he asked in a tremulous voice. "I've been scared wondering why the rush to Fort Wayne for a broken leg."

Sobbing, I told him, "They don't think he's going to make it. Most of his bones are broken. His legs, arms, collarbones, ribs. All of them. Some even broke before he was born."

Shocked, his mother cried, "How can that be?"

"He has a rare bone disease," I told them, and as I reached for the book on my bed stand, I realized that Dr. Burnes had left it to help me tell the heart-wrenching news to Dick and the rest of our family.

Chapter Two

In my hospital room, the blinds were tightly drawn. Yet bright slivers of sun filtered through the cracks and spilled gently on the white seersucker cover on my bed. Outside, a warm and beautiful April day was unfolding. A day when tulips would surely pop their heads out of the rich dark soil, and robins would busily build their nests.

Around the bed next to mine, a curtain was drawn, but from behind it, I heard the sounds of a suckling infant and a mother's cooing. Such sweet sounds. But for me, wrenching sounds that made me remember and started me crying again.

Peering curiously around the curtain, a young woman asked, "Is something wrong?"

I sobbed. "They took my baby away."

Making a soothing sound, she smiled. "Don't worry. They'll bring him back when he gets hungry. They've brought mine in twice already, and he was born just a few hours ago!"

Gently, she caressed her baby's tiny fingers and kissed the top of his head.

Were my baby's fingers broken? I wondered. Would they hurt if I was able to touch them? "My baby isn't here," I told her. "He was transferred to a Fort Wayne hospital because something is wrong with his bones."

"Oh, I'm sorry. I didn't know," she said and quickly popped back behind the curtain.

My eyes were closed even though I was wide-awake when a nurse came moments later to get the young woman's baby, so their quickly exchanged whispers behind the curtain did not escape me.

Moments later, Dr. Burnes arrived on his rounds. With feigned cheerfulness, he said, "Gemma, how would you like to go home?" Before I could reply, he looked directly at the drawn curtain around the other bed and said, "I think you'd feel better if you were out of here, don't you?"

I nodded yes.

In his best bedside manner, he continued, "I phoned Dick. He promised to take good care of you if I let you go home. I also phoned the doctors in Fort Wayne." He hesitated, then murmured, "I'm sorry." And my heart sank once more. "They hold little or no hope for your baby. He's the most severe case of osteogenesis imperfecta congenita that they've ever seen. Besides all the fractures, they say his skull is dangerously paper-thin."

The lump in my throat hurt so badly, I couldn't speak.

"I'm sorry," he repeated. "I'll call you. We'll talk again in a few days. In the meantime, the Fort Wayne doctors have promised to keep you posted several times a day on the baby's condition."

When Dick and I arrived at his parents' home, the family appeared to already be in mourning. The only exception was two-year-old Cathy who came running to me, smiling and begging for a big kiss and hug before I was whisked upstairs to our darkened bedroom. After Dick had dutifully tucked me into bed, I asked, "Have you said anything to Cathy yet?"

"I told her the baby was sick, and that I wasn't sure when we were going to bring him home," he said, choking back tears. "I thought you'd be better able to explain it to her . . . about the broken bones, I mean."

"We'll tell her about that only if we have to," I said. "Only if he does get to come home." For Cathy, who had just popped into the bedroom, I emphasized the positive. "Your little brother's name is Michael William. He has big blue eyes, blond hair, and looks just like Daddy!"

"Mikey," she giggled as she nestled close to me.

"Yes, let's call him Mikey," I said, feeling for the first time that our little son was a person and not just a horrible description in a medical textbook.

"Where's Mikey?" she asked with a frown.

"Mikey's hurt. The doctors at the hospital are taking care of him."

"Oh," she said, seemingly satisfied with my simple explanation, "Mikey's hurt."

Stifling the sobs that were bubbling in my throat, I drew her closer and let the feelings for my hurt baby pour out to her.

Downstairs, people were coming and going, tiptoeing, and talking in whispers. *They're having a wake, and the baby's not even dead yet*, I thought bitterly. We've got to stop this. We need to pray and think positive thoughts.

After two days of isolation in our bedroom, I couldn't stand it any longer, so I persuaded Dick to help me down the stairs so I could talk with the Fort Wayne doctors on the only phone available instead of having their bulletins relayed to me upstairs. I also needed to resume as normal a life as I could as soon as possible so we could move into our own home as planned.

Relieved to see me bouncing back so fast, Dick helped me down the stairs and helped me to settle on a sofa close to the phone and TV. As soon as I was settled, he turned the television on to a program about the opening of the baseball season. However, it turned out that the show was not only about major league baseball, but about Little League as well. Before us on the screen, there suddenly appeared scores of healthy, robust little boys running, swinging bats, and throwing balls. A strange strangled sound came from my husband, and someone quickly turned off the TV. That's all I remember, except for the dream I had that night about happy, healthy little boys running and playing baseball.

True to their promise, a pediatrician and an orthopedist from the Indiana hospital phoned us several times a day the first week. Mike was eating well, the pediatrician said, and other than the broken bones, seemed fairly healthy. The orthopedist's reports were more dire. He said that Mike had been put in a body cast and was being handled with extreme care. He stressed the severity of our baby's condition by telling us that the hospital's Catholic chaplain had been called in to baptize him. Coming from a large Catholic family, I knew that a hurried baptism in the hospital was a sure sign that death was near.

"Do you know that I still haven't seen my baby? You should have told us you were having him baptized. We would have come," I half-cried, half-scolded. "We're coming to see him right now, we need to hold him before it's too late," I finished.

"I don't think it's a good idea to see him, to get attached to him. And you certainly can't hold him. He's much too fragile," he cautioned.

"We're coming," I firmly insisted and hung up.

When we arrived at the hospital, we were led to a room set apart from the newborn nursery. It was a large room with a standard-sized crib with a big sign on it that read "FRAGILE, HANDLE WITH CARE." In the center of the huge-looking bed was a little mite of six pounds, encased in a plaster cast from his armpits to his toes. Only the diaper area was left uncasted.

From the puckered little face, alert blue eyes peered at us.

"Hi, we're your mommy and daddy," I said, taking his hand and feeling the immediate response of little fingers curling around mine. From the other side of the bed, Dick said hello and got a similar reaction. For a long time, we stayed in that position as the three of us attempted to connect. We'd been warned not to try to pick him up, so we stroked his silky hair, kissed his sweet lips, told him we loved him, and tried to bond with him in every possible way.

On the way home, I kept exclaiming, "He's so cute, as cute as any baby! And he looks healthy and normal, not like someone who's about to die! I thought he'd look different after everything Dr. Burnes and the other doctors have told us."

"He is cute," Dick agreed. "And I don't think he looks as sick as they say he is either."

Several days after our hospital visit, we moved into our newly decorated house where the crib and baby things had been readied with so much anticipation. Having sensed a small but definite change in the doctors' daily reports, we decided to wait a while before removing and storing the baby items. The doctors' tones were still cautious, yet different—more optimistic. "He's doing surprisingly well," they said. "If he continues this way, you're going to have to find alternative care. We can't keep him in the hospital indefinitely."

"There won't be any need to find alternative care," I said. "We're going to bring him home where he belongs."

"You can't do that," the doctor objected.

"Oh yes, we can!" I replied. He's *our* baby, isn't he?"

Chapter Three

The doctors had warned us to come for Mike with plenty of protective pillows. So with the backseat of the car equipped with a baby car bed surrounded by plump pillows, we headed for Fort Wayne. At the hospital, we barely had time to plant a kiss on our baby's forehead before instructions about handling him and about his formula began.

As the experienced baby nurse picked Mike up off the hospital bed to place him onto the large pillow that she would use to carry him, I noticed that the back of his head had changed from round to very flat since our last visit, and I cried, "My god, what happened to his head?"

Avoiding my eyes, the nurse said, "The doctors told you that his skull is very soft, didn't they?"

A bit confused, I replied, "Well, yes, but . . ."

"His skull being so soft and the fact that he's been on his back for two weeks shaped it that way," the nurse said. "I'm sorry."

"Couldn't you have put him on his side now and then to avert this?"

"We had orders to move him as little as possible so as not to fracture him."

Bewildered, I said, "But nearly all of his body is in a cast! Was he breaking inside the cast?"

"His arms are exposed," she pointed out. "Even so, I wish I could have done more for him. But I've never—none of us have ever seen, much less handled, a breakable baby. We were told not to move him unless absolutely necessary, and we did what we were told."

Dick and I looked at each other in dismay and said no more.

Seeing our reaction, her professional veneer softened. "I'm sorry. I really am. About everything."

After an appointment had been made to come back for x-rays and to possibly have the cast removed, the same nurse accompanied us to the car carrying Mike on a large pillow like an exquisite china doll. With great care, she placed him in the padded car bed and hastily wished us good luck.

During the long drive home, Dick drove slowly, easing our old car gently around potholes and bumps while I sat on the edge of the backseat, holding my wide-eyed baby's hand.

At home, Dick's parents and Cathy were waiting our arrival; and as soon as we pulled the car up alongside the house, the door swung open, and Cathy came running to see her little brother. With one swift motion, her grandmother restrained her.

Once inside, Dick and I lifted Mike out of the car bed and placed him in the waiting crib. When they saw his flattened head and cumbersome body cast, a sad, agonized look passed like an ominous cloud across the faces of his grandparents.

Dick tried to comfort them. "He's going to be okay. Gemma and I will take good care of him."

"We know you will," his mother said gently. "We'll help too anytime you need us."

This initial response from the two people who loved our children more than anything else should have alerted us how others would react to Mike, but it didn't. We were too concerned with the immediate problem of guarding him against bodily injury.

Later, when Cathy had gone to spend the night with her grandparents to afford us some undisturbed time to get used to caring for Mike, Dick and I finally had a chance to take a closer look at our little boy. What we saw appalled us.

Gross hospital neglect was glaringly apparent. The folds of Mike's neck were crusted with dried, soured milk; his scalp was yellow and flaky. Feces smeared the edges of his cast in the diaper area, and the odor of urine was overpowering. All I could do was look at our baby and cry until Dick brought me a basin of warm water and a soft washcloth. Then, working together, we cautiously moved him and sponged the exposed areas of his small six-pound body and the offensive portion of his cast, slathered a mildly scented baby lotion into every crease, then covered him with a clean blanket. In no time, he was fast asleep.

That first night when he woke up for his feeding, I was petrified, and my hands trembled when I tried to change his diaper without help. But I knew I had to do it; I wasn't about to neglect him the way the hospital staff had. So with tears rolling down my cheeks, I changed him even though I was afraid to move his little legs in the plaster cast. No one had been able to assure me that he wouldn't break while casted, and with horror, I remembered how he had fractured while softly cushioned in my womb.

Even after he had been changed and fed, I continued to sit by his padded bed in the dark of night while the phrases in my head alternated from "How can I take care of this child?" to "Oh, God, please help me take care of him."

I did a lot of crying those first days and weeks. We had so many questions for which there were either no answers or confusing and conflicting ones. When we asked how osteogenesis imperfecta had happened to Mike, we heard "It wasn't anything you did or didn't do. It's simply a quirk of nature. It couldn't happen again in the same family, so don't worry. Go ahead, have other children." Another answer to the same question was "There are known cases that appear to be passed down several generations in some families. Perhaps it would be a good idea not to have other children until we know more about it."

When we wanted to know how many children were similarly affected, we were told, "Osteogenesis imperfecta is very rare, and most of the children with the severe form that Mike has don't survive past their first year. Therefore, there are few statistics about those who do survive." Or "A number of children improve greatly during adolescence. Our best estimates are that there are at least three hundred known cases in the U.S."

When Dr. Burnes called or came over to see how we were doing, I mainly asked him baby-care questions, to which he frequently replied, "Did you ask the Fort Wayne doctors? What did *they* say?"

I had no faith in the Fort Wayne doctors and nurses after the way they had treated Mike, and I told him so. In response, he said he'd send the local county health nurse over to see if she could help or advise us on how to care for Mike. "Perhaps she'd be helpful," he said, "until we could find a home for crippled children [his words for an institution] that would take Mike."

Marcile Spayd, the county health nurse, was a middle-aged lady who had never married or had children. Mostly, she tended to the elderly who were confined to wheelchairs or were chronically ill. Some of her other duties were giving inoculations and eye tests to schoolchildren. Never in any of her lifetime experiences as a county health nurse had she seen anyone with osteogenesis imperfecta, let alone a baby with an estimated thirty to fifty healed or healing fractures. Nevertheless, she came to us when Dr. Burnes asked.

Her chunky-heeled shoes and her staid navy blue skirt and coat were her uniform, and her manner was gruff and businesslike. The first time I met her, my reaction wasn't very favorable, especially when she began talking about institutionalizing Mike before she had even had a chance to see him. "You certainly can't have other children around him, especially an active two-year-old," she said, echoing Dr. Burnes's words. "It would be too dangerous. I'm told that a slight bump could cause a broken arm or leg. Rough and tumble play could fracture his skull, or worse. If you decide to keep him home, you will definitely have to place Cathy in another household . . . with her grandparents perhaps."

I gasped. "Give up Cathy! Never!"

Her voice reaching a higher octave of final authority, she said, "Then you'll have to place the baby."

Stubbornly, I replied, "I'm not giving up either one of them!"

Softening somewhat, she said, "You don't have to decide right now. Talk to Dick about it. Then we'll discuss it again. Now, as long as I'm here, why don't you show me how you've been caring for him."

Still fuming at the idea of giving up either one of our children, I took her to Mike's crib, where I demonstrated how I had learned to slip a soiled diaper off and replace it with a fresh one without barely moving him. I showed her how his head had flattened while in the hospital and how I was trying to correct it by propping him on his side against a plump pillow. When she asked how I bathed and dressed him, I told her about the method Dick and I had developed for washing him and showed her the loose little shirts with the opening down the front that I had sewn for him to wear instead of using pullover shirts.

Her voice tinged with admiration *and* relief, she told me, "You're doing real well. Maybe you won't need me after all."

By then, my earlier resentment of her had vanished. Telling her what I was doing for Mike and getting her approval had been a great shot in the arm for me. It wasn't much, but it was the kind of support I so desperately needed. So without hesitation, I said, "Please come back. I'm sure I'm going to need a lot of help and advice."

Seeming pleased, she said, "I'm sure you already know more about this disease than I do. But if you want me to come, I will."

And she did. I don't know how she knew, but she always seemed to pop in when I needed her most. I remember once she came over right after I had heard a terrible cracking sound while dressing Mike. "It sounded like a pencil snapping," I told her. "But it must have been an arm or leg."

Her businesslike face began to crumble before she turned away. "That's probably what it was," she murmured. "Let's take him to the emergency room to find out."

When she learned that we had no medical insurance that would cover Mike's fractures, she immediately set about helping us to apply for state aid for crippled children. Once it was approved, she was the one who drove Mike and me to Lima, Ohio, to meet his new orthopedist, Dr. Howard Kingsbury, so Dick wouldn't have to lose time away from work.

What I appreciated most, though, was that after her first visit, Ms. Spayd never again mentioned sending either of our children to live away from home. Instead, she did all she could to help us keep them both.

After several months, Dr. Burnes also stopped talking about finding a home that would take Mike. That suited us just fine since we had known the instant we'd seen our baby in the oversized bed at the Fort Wayne hospital that, God willing, we would bring him home, care for him, and love him for as along as he was in our trust.

Chapter Four

Mike's first year proved to be a difficult and lonely one. The difficulties included knowing little about the disorder that affected him and not being able to find anyone who *did* know what was in store for us. Emotionally, we were in a dark abyss, crying to be heard and yearning to be told that Mike would be okay.

But our cries went unheard, our hopes unrealized. Our child was a rarity, an oddity, the only one in town ever diagnosed with osteogenesis imperfecta. There was absolutely no one who could tell us "We know how you feel, we've been there too."

When Mike cried, I thought my heart would break from wanting to pick him up and hold him close. But dutifully, I remembered all the warnings and tried to comfort him as he lay in his crib. Other times, when I suspected that he might be hurting from a new fracture, I felt totally inadequate because I didn't know how to ease his pain.

The word about Mike's condition had obviously gotten around in our new neighborhood. Neighbors stared curiously whenever we left the house, but none of them ever came over to welcome us and our children. Friends who had previously brought their toddlers over to play with Cathy stayed away, concerned that their active children might inadvertently hurt Mike.

I was raised the twelfth child in a fun-loving family of thirteen children, and I'd always been surrounded by what seemed like armies of people who shared one another's joys and burdens. Now in a strange town with all my family hundreds of miles away on the East Coast, my support system had dwindled down to a precious few. Dick's parents and his younger brother, Jim, were tremendously supportive, and they *did* help a lot with Cathy, but they had jobs and weren't always available to help when Mike fractured and had to be rushed to the doctor's office or emergency room.

When, several months after Mike's birth, my mother came to visit from Connecticut with my brother Pete and my sister Gerry and her husband, Edwin, I realized more than ever just how nervous everyone was about our baby's condition. Even my mother, who had held and nurtured countless babies, was fearful of helping me diaper and bathe my child.

Standing by Mike's crib one day during their visit, I was bursting to say, "Isn't he sweet!" like any mother would, but I remained silent and kept my maternal pride to myself. Even though I now regularly focused my attention on Mike's quick blue eyes, his easy smile, and the small fluff of blond on his head rather than on his flattened head and crooked limbs, I sensed that it was too soon for them to see him as I did.

They weren't ready to give me the kind of reassurance I craved. They could only offer me their prayers. "I'll pray for a miracle for Mike. That's all I can do," Mother said as they were leaving.

Wanting to believe as strongly as she did, I replied wryly, "I hope God hears you."

My own optimism about prayer was quickly waning. Most of the time, I questioned and begged rather than prayed. "Why our baby, Lord? Why us? What did we do? Why is Mike being punished? Why are we? Haven't I always tried to be good? Haven't I been faithful?" Or "Please, God, make my son healthy. Let him sit, walk, and play like other children. All you have to do is snap your fingers, and his pain and suffering will be gone. Please, God!"

When I posed some of these questions in letters to my eldest sister, Fernande, a Roman Catholic nun, her response was usually "Keep praying. Have faith. Someday God will let you know the reason."

Someday seemed too remote. I needed help *now* so that I could bring normalcy back into our lives. Our nights out as a couple had virtually stopped because it was so hard to find anyone willing to babysit Mike. Other than Dick's family, few came to visit. I was so wrapped up in caring for Mike, I didn't even realize that Cathy was spending too much time playing alone in her room. At least, I thought she was playing alone until

I passed her bedroom door one day and overheard her talking. Standing quietly by the door, I listened as she engaged in a lengthy conversation with two individuals named Tex and Ernie.

Approaching her, I quizzed, "Cathy, who are Tex and Ernie?"

With wide-eyed innocence, she explained, "Ernie's my pretend brother, and Tex is my pretend friend."

"But you have a real brother," I objected.

"Mikey can't play," she replied mournfully.

Having lost nearly all her playmates and having been warned time and time again not to go anywhere near her baby brother, Cathy had invented herself an imaginary friend and brother to play with. Getting down on my knees, I scooped her up and hugged her while I silently rebuked myself for not having known how lonely she was.

Following the advice of doctors and other professionals, we had isolated each child from the other to avoid the possibility of fractures. Now common sense told me that this had been a useless precaution since Mike sometimes fractured spontaneously while alone in his own bed. That evening, Dick and I talked it over and decided it was time to put an end to this senseless segregation.

Reading books together had always been a special activity that Cathy and I had enjoyed but that I had pitifully neglected since Mike's birth. Realizing that reading would be a safe yet fun way that the two of us could spend time with Mike, I began reading to Cathy while sitting near his crib. Soon, much to her delight, Mike began cooing whenever he heard her reciting the many stories she had memorized. Once she was included, Cathy would come to me with a pile of books under her arm whenever Mike was fussy, and with her brown curls bouncing with big-sister importance, she'd ask, "You want me to read to him, Mommy?"

These special times together also gave me a chance to share information with Cathy about Mike's disability a bit at a time and in ways that she could understand. Whenever he had a fracture and had a limb in a splint or cast, I'd wrap her baby doll's leg or arm to demonstrate how it was needed to support the hurting limb. Or I'd show her how to diaper her doll without grabbing the baby's ankles the way it was normally done but, rather, by placing her hand gently under the doll's lower back to lift her buttocks. These special instructions were effective ways of teaching her that we had to be extra careful with our baby. The day I overheard her asking Mike through his crib bars, "Poor baby with broken legs, don't you wish you had wings so you could fly?" I knew that she also understood that he wouldn't be able to walk.

Our success allowing Mike and Cathy to be together encouraged us to try expanding our own relationship with Mike—a relationship that had, until now, been more vocal than physical.

Gradually, and with great care, we began lifting him out of his crib. For short periods of time, we gave him the luxury of our big bed where he could see the world from a different perspective and where, with supervision, Cathy could snuggle up close to him. Dick often sang silly little songs to Cathy, and now feeling closer to Mike, he sang them for him too. In response, Mike gave us the first sound of his laughter.

These successful experiences made us braver, and before long, we were propping Mike up in a reclining position. When we discovered just weeks before his first birthday that I was pregnant, I cried at first because I didn't know how I would be able to care for a third child. Then out of necessity, I put my tears and fears aside and, with Dick's help, got down to the business of accelerating Mike's rehabilitation into the real world. With a toddler and two babies in the house, there would be no more time for Mike's long, tedious sponge baths. So when he was not encumbered with casts, we began immersing him in a bit of warm water in a small plastic tub that we lined with a thin pad so he wouldn't slide. The results were amazing. Mike loved kicking and splashing in the water, and though we didn't realize it then, his time spent in the tub was very good for strengthening his bones.

Slowly, but steadily, he progressed; and by the time his first birthday rolled around, his upper body was much stronger, and he could hold his head up unassisted. To celebrate, we bought him a bright yellow canvas teeter-babe chair that was tip proof and had springs to make it bounce.

On the day he turned one, Cathy jumped up and down with glee as we sat him in his brand-new chair. In turn, Mike gurgled and laughed, and his eyes shone with delight. For the first time, he was seeing the world on an even keel, and he seemed quite pleased with what he saw.

Chapter Five

Not long after Mike's first birthday, we bought a four-bedroom house with a large backyard in the neighborhood where Dick had grown up and where his parents still lived. It proved to be a good move for us and for Cathy, who immediately made friends with Sharon, the little girl next door.

Also fun for Mike and Cathy were the daily visits from Dick's old family dog Shorty. Part German shepherd and part mongrel, Shorty had quickly figured out a shortcut alongside a creek that flowed past fields, an apple orchard, and our house and his. Like clockwork, he would meander into our yard every morning, the same as an employee reporting for work, and find himself a spot to snooze until the children came out to play.

If the weather was good enough for Mike to be on the porch in his teeter-babe or playpen, Shorty would appoint himself his guardian by snarling fiercely at anyone who dared come near him. He seemed to sense that Mike needed his protection more than Cathy did; he seldom budged from his side, even when I was nearby. Once Mike was brought back into the house, relieving Shorty of his self-appointed duty, he would wander off to find Cathy and her friend to see what they were doing. Then at dusk, he'd head back home again down his path along the creek.

Our new neighborhood was friendlier than the last in many ways. Maybe it was because most of the people who lived there knew Dick's family, or maybe it was because they saw me growing bigger with our third child and felt sorry for me in light of Mike's condition. But every now and then, the elderly lady two doors down would bring me cut peonies from her garden, and others showered us with their vegetable garden excess. Having Dick's parents near was also a big plus since hardly an evening went by that they didn't come over to play with the children or help bathe them and put them to bed.

And so it was into this much happier environment that Cindy was born on Thanksgiving Day 1957. Weighing in at seven pounds, she had a perfectly rounded head, a cute little nose, and straight arms and legs. After Dr. Burnes had assured me over and over again that she was perfect, I took time out to say a prayer of thanksgiving for the beautiful, healthy baby that had appropriately been given to us on the day set aside for giving thanks.

Though I hadn't voiced it to anyone but Dick, I had been terrified throughout my pregnancy of having another baby with osteogenesis imperfecta, and I'd been plagued with bad dreams about it.

In one particularly scary dream, I had spent the night opening dresser drawers only to find every one of them occupied by an OI baby with a huge deformed head and grotesquely crooked limbs. I had awakened from that dream shaken and positive that it meant that the baby I was carrying and, any other babies after that, would be born with OI. What a relief it was to know that my interpretation had been wrong.

The response to Cindy's birth was the exact opposite of Mike's. This time, friends and relatives came in droves to examine our baby and to exclaim over her beauty. It was as if they were breathing a collective sigh of relief, not only because this child was healthy, but because they were being given a second chance to make up for the way they had reacted to Mike.

My mother, who had flown in from the East Coast to help, picked Cindy up every time she let out a peep. Cradling her in her arms, she crooned in her French Canadian tongue about Cindy's beautiful long eyelashes and her little cheeks, pink as roses. Her chants always ended with the same exclamation, "Quel belle poupee!" meaning, "What a beautiful doll!"

Secretly, I felt the same about Cindy. Holding her close in my arms the way I hadn't been able to hold Mike was pure delight. Often, I caught myself rubbing her perfectly rounded head and feeling her strong sturdy limbs with fingers that danced at the wonder of her. These were feelings that I'd had at Cathy's birth—normal feelings that most new mothers take for granted, but that now felt rare to me after eighteen long months of trying to avoid touching a child whose bones were as fragile as glass.

When Mike was close by, I had to make a determined effort not to rave about Cindy the way everyone else was doing. And finally, I had to have a quiet talk with my aging mother about the way *she* was acting.

When Cathy had been only a few months old, she and I had gone to Maine to stay with my mother while Dick's ship was at sea. It had been during that cold and difficult winter after my father's death, and alone in the big house that had once been so full, that my mother and I had learned to share our most intimate feelings with each other.

Now my mother nodded in silent agreement when I respectfully reminded her that she had never fawned over any of her own children the way she was fawning over Cindy. Instead, she had always tried to focus her attention on our individual talents and attributes. After our talk, Mother had tried hard to spread her energies among all three of our children. Once or twice, she had even summoned the courage to hold Mike and bathe him or feed him so she could get some kind of physical connection with him.

Though she still spoke of praying for a miracle, my mother's parting words were of a different sort this time. "Frankly," she said, "I don't think you should have any more children. Why don't you ask the priest for permission to use something?"

"Ma, I can't believe I'm hearing that from you!" I cried, shocked. This kind of advice was so completely out of character for her.

Smiling, my devout Catholic mother retorted, "If I'd known about things like that, half of you children wouldn't be here."

Being the twelfth child, I cried, "Thank God you didn't!"

Dick and I had decided long before my mother spoke of it to ask our pastor for permission to use birth control even though we knew it was against the teachings of the church. Because of our special circumstances, we felt sure that we would be granted a dispensation.

Our silver-haired pastor gave a practiced gasp from behind the little screen in the confessional when I made my request. "No no no, that's impossible!" he hissed with disapproval. "The church won't allow it no matter what the circumstances."

Crushed, I left the confessional. When Dick got the same response, we determined to try to follow the church's teachings by following what they called the rhythm method, which consisted of a time of abstinence every month when conception was most likely. It failed miserably. Several months later, I was pregnant again, but suffered a miscarriage at the end of the first trimester.

Later on, our parish had a seminar on the rhythm method for couples wishing to limit their families the approved way. The seminar was conducted by a husband-and-wife team, who were also a doctor and a nurse. At the end of the presentation, when they welcomed questions from the audience, someone asked, "How many children do you folks have?" They answered, "Ten."

Grabbing my arm, Dick murmured, "This is a bunch of baloney. Let's get out of here." From that moment on, we decided to do what *we* thought best about limiting *our* family.

Finding our own way was becoming a fact of life for us since there was no one apparently equipped or willing to challenge the consequences of living with OI. Another difficult choice we eventually had to make had to do with the treatment of Mike's fractures.

Most of the time when Mike broke a bone and had to be driven thirty miles to the orthopedist's office, the x-rays revealed what we already knew, that he had a fracture. But the broken limb, usually an arm or a leg, was never reset and seldom casted, but was wrapped instead with an Ace bandage or put in a sling to provide support. From the start, we'd been told, "We're sorry, there's little else we can do. Trying to set the bone would only cause more damage."

Aware that the trip, the handling, and the frequent x-rays were becoming more traumatic for Mike than the fractures themselves, we decided to splint and wrap his limbs ourselves whenever we suspected a simple hairline fracture. For the more severe fractures, we continued to rely on his orthopedist.

The months immediately following Cindy's birth were hectic, but happy. Dick was working on a heavy construction job, but no matter how tired he was at the end of the day, he always spent time playing with the children or helping me with the chores I hadn't finished. Sometimes, weeks went by without seeing or talking to another adult other than Dick and his parents. For that reason, my evenings with them were very precious to me.

Dick's dad wasn't the same type of personality that my own father had been, so I didn't really look at him as a substitute dad, but I did have a nice buddylike relationship with him. He and Dick were very close, and the best thing about their closeness was that they were willing to include me in it. Sometimes, when Dick was caring for the children, especially

Mike, his dad and I would beam our mutual pride and admiration across the room to each other. Or he'd look at his former football player, boxing-champion son and whisper, "He's good with them, isn't he?" Other times, when the children did or said something cute, he and I often erupted into simultaneous laughter.

That spring, Memorial Day had been a happy one picnicking with the children on the banks of the Maumee River. Dick and his dad had fished and listened to the Indianapolis 500 car race on the radio, and his mother and I had fixed lunch, then lazed on blankets while the children napped. That evening, as usual, Mom and Dad had helped us bathe and put the children to bed before going on home. After they had left, we'd collapsed into bed and were sleeping soundly until the phone's persistent ringing had jarred us awake. Mom's voice, shaky but controlled, summoned Dick to come over quickly. Dad had suddenly taken ill, and a doctor had been called.

Misdiagnosed at first as having a case of indigestion, Dad wasn't admitted to the hospital. Several days later, suffering from confusion, fever, and a stiff neck, he was taken to a Lima, Ohio, hospital with a tentative spinal meningitis diagnosis. There, he was placed in isolation, and those of us who had been exposed to the infectious disease were inoculated. When a neurologist finally examined him, the diagnosis was changed again, this time to a brain aneurysm. After endless hours of brain surgery, we were told that the operation appeared successful, yet Dad never regained consciousness; and several weeks later, he died at the age of fifty-one due to complications of pneumonia.

Dick, his mother, and brother were brokenhearted. I was devastated and disillusioned. Throughout Dad's illness, I had prayed that he would be spared and allowed to stay with us, but again, my prayers and supplications had been ignored. One of our most generous and loving supporters was gone; our circle of support irrevocably broken.

Dick's brother Jim and his wife, Mary, returned to his army post after the funeral. And his mom, who was overwhelmed with grief and had to deal with unpaid hospital bills and sudden widowhood, needed time to heal and sort out her own life. Though we made a determined effort to keep her at the center of our lives, we all knew that our family life could never be the same again. Thank goodness for the children who kept us too busy to mope and who brought cheer no matter how dark the times.

By then, Mike was full of mischief. Bright and with a lot of time on his hands to dream up the things that two—and three-year-olds normally do, he improvised his inability to act by having Cindy carry out the deeds. At ten months, Cindy was walking; at a year old, she was running and climbing. If Mike wanted cookies from the cookie jar on the kitchen counter, she'd push a chair over and hop up and get him some. When he fancied petting (teasing) the cat, she'd grab it by the tail and place it on his lap. He directed their activities; she carried them out. These joint adventures resulted in all kinds of minor disasters that should have gotten both of them in hot water. Yet from the moment she could talk, Cindy didn't blame Mike, but instead took it upon herself to defend him. Her beautiful blue eyes welling with tears and her lower lip trembling, she'd confess, "Mike didn't do it! I did!"

Technically, she was right. But knowing that Mike instigated most of their deeds, how could we punish her?

Having been there before him, Cathy had to be taught about Mike's frailties and how to cope with them. But not Cindy, whose symbiotic relationship with Mike appeared to be based on their mutual desires rather than on Mike's differences. Because they always did things together, it soon became apparent to Cindy that Mike was being singled out for special favors by friends and relatives. "How come Aunt Mabel gave Mike a quarter but didn't give me one?" she'd question in an I-want-to-know voice. Or "Why is Mike getting toys? It's not his birthday!"

Cathy had voiced her resentment about the way some of the older relatives showered small gifts or money on "poor little Mike," but she'd never done it as forcefully as Cindy did. Or maybe she just hadn't been as persistent.

Hoping the girls would understand what motivated the gift giving, I told them, "I guess they think Mike is special."

Cathy nodded, "Yeah, 'cause he can't walk."

As if she was discovering this difference for the first time, Cindy thought about it for a moment, then said, "Yeah, I guess." Then with her hands on her hips and a toss of her head, she added, "But I'm special too!"

And indeed, she was.

Chapter Six

"Here I come to save the day!" Mike sang as he flexed his muscles like Mighty Mouse, one of his TV superheroes. In his mind, he imagined himself strong and full of the vitality needed to do great physical deeds. For Christmas and his birthdays, the number one item on his wish list was always a can of spinach—the magic stuff that propelled his other TV hero, the gravely voiced Popeye, to victory over overwhelming odds. Catering to his fantasies, we gave him all the spinach he asked for. But neither the spinach nor our prayers for miracles had any effect whatsoever on the ravages of OI.

At age four, Mike was barely the size of a one-year-old, and his arms and legs had grown more crooked and deformed by the numerous fractures he'd suffered since birth. He couldn't dress himself or go to the bathroom unassisted, but he could scoot on the floor on his little bottom when the coast was clear. Otherwise, he got around from place to place in his father's arms or mine.

He did, however, have a vocabulary that far surpassed that of most four-year-olds, as well as an extraordinary ability to figure out how to surmount his limitations. Sometimes I wondered how he knew so much; he was so sheltered. Once when both his arms were in slings and one leg was in a cast, he showed his resourcefulness by using his five remaining toes to play with his toys and also became quite proficient at turning the pages of books with his chin.

"He's a spunky kid all right," his orthopedist said when we told him about these accomplishments. Until then, Dr. Kingsbury had tended to Mike's fractures but had never discussed any other treatments. This time, though, he had a pensive look on his face as he worked to remove Mike's cast. When done, he turned to us and said, "I know a doctor in Chicago who might be able to straighten Mike's legs. His name is Dr. Harold Sofield. I was a resident at Shriners Hospital for Crippled Children when he developed his rodding technique."

Surprised, I said, "But I thought nothing could be done for Mike's bones. At least, that's what everyone's been telling us for over four years."

"Even in the orthopedic community, not everyone is familiar with the procedure. Generally, we don't mention it until we know the child will . . ." His voice trailed, and embarrassed, he looked at Mike, who was still sitting on the casting table.

From the time he was born, the professionals who had cared for Mike had openly discussed the rarity of his diagnosis and his medical prognosis in front of him. Now that he was older and much smarter, we had asked them not to engage in this practice. Dr. Kingsbury, who had been about to say that they didn't mention the Sofield procedure until they were sure the child would live, had caught himself just in time. His face was red, and he cleared his throat and continued, "As I was saying about the rodding surgery—"

"Yes, tell us more," I cut in eagerly.

"I haven't done a rodding procedure since leaving Shriners, so I wouldn't want to attempt it. But if you're interested, I'll contact Dr. Sofield."

"What exactly is rodding surgery?" Dick asked, trying not to sound too elated.

"The procedure involves placing a steel rod inside the bone to strengthen it and to reduce fractures."

Mike's ears perked up. "Steel rods? In *my* bones!" he exclaimed.

"Whoa, hold on," Dr. Kingsbury cautioned. "We're only talking about it. Maybe it can be done, maybe it can't."

"Tell us what we have to do to get in to see Dr. Sofield. I don't care how expensive it is. Whatever the cost, we'll find a way," Dick said.

Dr. Kingsbury smiled broadly. "You won't have to pay a cent if you qualify," he said. "You'll have the best bone man in the country and the best hospital care at no cost."

"That's incredible! How do we qualify?" I interjected.

"All you have to do is locate a member of the Shriner organization in your hometown who is willing to sponsor Mike and guide you through the application process," he said. "I'll do the rest."

On the way home from Lima that day, Dick and I were bubbling over just thinking about all the possibilities rodding offered. "Maybe it's the miracle we've been praying for," I whispered.

"Maybe," Dick said with a catch in his voice.

From the backseat came the sound of Mike's voice humming, "Here I come to save the day!" as he too considered the possibilities of rodding. It was so apropos, and we both burst out laughing.

In no time at all, we located a businessman who was a Shriner willing to sponsor Mike for admittance to Shriners Hospital. Dr. Kingsbury made the necessary consultations with Dr. Sofield, and before we could think the entire matter through, we were headed for Chicago.

Though we had often spoken about Mike's hospitalization during the weeks that preceded his admittance, the full impact of his leaving our care for months of surgery at a distant hospital didn't really hit home until we were actually on our way. Mike hadn't been hospitalized since the weeks that had followed his birth. Remembering vividly the way he had been neglected then now became a grave concern. Another worry was that Mike had never been away overnight other than to his grandmother's house. Nor had he ever been left with anyone other than family for more than a few hours. Yet he had assured us during our frequent talks that he could handle going away if it meant coming back with steel in his legs. But what does a four-year-old, who has always been the focus of attention, know about loneliness?

Since most of the young patients at Shriners came long distances for their surgery and other treatments, and since most of them attended school classes at the hospital on weekdays, it had been suggested to us that we visit only on weekends since the trip for us was a five-hundred-mile roundtrip. This was agreeable, but the hospital's policy that parents could not be present during surgery was not.

Though there were a number of reasons for this policy, the main one was that surgery was sometimes scheduled, then canceled, and rescheduled if the child had a cold, fever, or other malady the day of surgery. We were told that it was unreasonable to expect parents to travel long distances only to have the surgery canceled at the last minute. Since we couldn't be there, we would be notified only after the surgery had been completed.

Logically, the explanations made sense. Emotionally, they did not. We had already filled out all sorts of information sheets about Mike's favorite foods, toys, likes, and dislikes. But if we weren't there, who would hold his hand and tell him not to be afraid as he was wheeled into surgery? Who would come to soothe him when he was hurting? Mike had been very quiet in the backseat of the car since kissing Cathy and Cindy a tearful good-bye. Was it fair to separate him from his faithful siblings for such a long time?

What if we were making a bad decision about surgery? Maybe his fragile bones wouldn't be able to hold the rods. Maybe he'd have to go through all that pain for nothing. And what if something went wrong? Would we be able to live with our decision?

By the time we pulled into the hospital parking lot, we were so overwhelmed with doubt, we were ready to turn around and take him home. But how could we deny him the promise of fewer fractures and the chance to have stronger, straighter legs? Shriners was the only hospital in the country that offered him that chance. So reluctantly, we stayed.

"Hi, Snicklefritz!" the renowned Dr. Sofield greeted Mike. "How are you?" He extended his hand to Mike, then to us. Sizing Mike up with kindly eyes, he said, "I understand you want rods in your legs."

"Yup," Mike replied happily.

"Well, then, you've come to the right place."

As if on cue, a candy striper appeared. "Why don't you go with this nice young lady," the genial doctor told Mike. "Take a tour of the place. See if it suits you."

Appearing suddenly panic-stricken, Mike turned to me for reassurance.

"Don't worry. We'll still be here when you get back," I promised.

The candy striper buckled him into a tiny wheelchair and wheeled him out the door. Once they were gone, Dr. Sofield told us that he had conferred with Dr. Kingsbury, had reviewed Mike's x-rays, and agreed that he was a good candidate for rodding. During the rodding procedures, he explained that, one surgery at a time, Mike's femurs, then his tibias, would be removed from his legs. The length of bone would be chopped up and strung back on a metal rod in shish kebab fashion and put back into place. Since Mike was so severely affected, rodding still wouldn't allow him to walk, but would definitely straighten his bones, provide strength, and minimize his fractures. Following each operation, the leg would remain in a cast for about eight weeks. During that time, Mike would remain in the hospital until the next phase of surgery. The entire process, he said, would probably take six or more months.

Following the rodding explanation, Dr. Sofield listed his credentials and, to reassure us, mentioned that it was likely that he had seen and operated on more OI patients than any other orthopedist and, therefore, would be glad to fill us in on some of the interesting as well as some of the other important aspects of the disorder. As he spoke, we soon realized that we had been told only the most basic facts. Fascinating to us was the information that many OI children looked alike and that there were children with the milder form of OI, known as OI tarda, who could walk and live near-normal lives. Hearing all this new information about OI was like cramming an entire course of Osteogenesis Imperfecta 101 in all at once.

After our interview with Dr. Sofield, the candy striper returned Mike so we could have time together to say good-bye. Both Dick and I took turns holding him on our laps for comforting hugs and words of love and encouragement. Then before we realized quite what was happening, a hospital worker came to escort us to the little boys' ward where the nursing staff was waiting for him.

As we walked down the long sterile hospital corridor to the ward, I felt Mike's arms tightening around my neck, and it felt as if he was squeezing my heart as well.

In the little boys' ward, a friendly, matronly nurse reached out for Mike and told him to bid us good-bye. I wanted to take him back and say, "No, thank you. I've changed my mind. Give him back." But already, the nurse was walking away from us and motioning us to leave. All at once, Mike howled, "I don't want to stay! I want to go home!"

Feeling like traitors, we hurried down the hallway with his wails echoing behind us and walked out the door, not daring to look back. In the car, Dick sat motionless, his big muscular hands clenching the steering wheel until his knuckles matched the whiteness of his face. Unshed tears welled in his eyes, and I turned from him to brush away my own tears.

Those first weeks without Mike were terribly lonely; we were so accustomed to his needs, his demands, his constant presence. In the beginning, our thoughts were constantly with him in Chicago, and every free moment was spent writing little notes and cards to cheer him up. The weekend after we were notified of his first surgery, we drove the five hundred miles to visit him.

He sported a large, bulky cast and seemed pale and listless the first time we visited. We carried an armload of gifts for him, but when he spotted us, he turned his face toward the wall and wouldn't look at us. When finally we were able to cajole him to turn around, we saw that he had been weeping silently. With big sorrowful eyes, he looked at us, and all at once, his chest heaved and out came a torrent of heart-wrenching sobs, between which he begged us to take him home. It wasn't until months later that we learned that Mike had overheard that another young patient had once been brought to the hospital and abandoned by his parents.

Leaving Mike at Shriners the first time had been difficult; the second time was pure torture. The sounds of his screams followed us all the way home and continued to haunt us for days. So much so that we dreaded going back. But surprisingly, the next time wasn't bad at all. Mike seemed his old self. Excitedly, he showed us the heap of toys he'd received after his second surgery and told us about some of the friends he'd made. And there were no more crying fits when we finally had to leave. So it was with much lighter hearts that we traveled home that day and on subsequent visits.

With the pains of separation behind us, we began to relax and enjoy the freedom of doing the normal things that families do. We visited friends, went to the movies, and did all the things we couldn't do when Mike was home. It felt so good being able to go out without everyone staring at us and feeling sorry for us. Sometimes my joy at being free of these encumbrances evoked guilty feelings, but not for long. *Enjoy it while you can*, I told myself. Another baby was due soon, and Mike too would be home before we knew it. Soon there would be four children to care for—three of them under the age of five.

On November 5 of that year, Mike came home proud of his straight legs, scars, and all. On November 9, the day after John Kennedy was elected president, our second son was born, weighing in at a healthy nine pounds. When one of the nurses asked me if we were naming him after Richard Nixon, the defeated candidate, I scoffed, "Of course not!" Then proudly, I told them, "We're naming him after his father and grandfather."

Chapter Seven

The weeks and months that followed Mike's return home from Shriners and Dickie's birth were filled with hope and joy. Our second son was a contented baby who seemed to have been born with a smile on his face. Cathy, who was six by then, loved to hold him and talk to him. In return, he rewarded her generously by being enraptured with the sound of her voice. At last, the void in Cathy's life—the expectation of a healthy little brother—had been filled.

At three, Cindy, who loved playing house, was thrilled to have a new baby to mother, as well as having Mike, her "pretend" husband, back home again.

Dick and I were ecstatic, not only at the birth of a healthy son, but also because we felt more secure about Mike's future now that he had steel rods in his legs.

In the Washington White House, the Kennedys reigned over Camelot. In the Geisman household, the new feeling of normalcy was enough for us. For the boys, what could have been more normal than the great American pastime of baseball?

During his long stay at the Chicago hospital, Mike had become a devoted Chicago Cubs fan who talked about nothing but baseball. This new interest created a strong bond between father and son, and they spent a great deal of their free time watching the televised games together.

It soon became obvious to all who knew him that, in his heart and mind, Mike was an athlete. With rare instinct, he seemed to know ahead of time what the coaches and players were going to do next or how they were going to get themselves out of a jam. Mike's head knew how to execute a game plan, but physically, he couldn't play it out. Dickie could, and before long, he was doing it for both of them.

From the moment he could stand up and hold a ball and clench a plastic Wiffle bat in his hands, Mike and Dad were teaching him how to wind up for a pitch or how and when to swing a bat. When the boys weren't playing baseball, Mike and Dad were talking about it, and Dickie was absorbing it. Before long, there was a threesome watching the televised games, assessing the major leaguers, recording batting averages, and collecting baseball cards.

The reduced number of spontaneous fractures in Mike's "rodded" legs and the trips to Chicago for his postsurgical checkups were the only reminders during those busy years that OI was still a part of our lives.

The trips to Chicago were always undertaken with much dread. The drive through rural Indiana took approximately three hours, but it always took another nerve-wracking two or three hours of hectic driving through heavy traffic to get to the suburb of Oak Park, where the hospital was located. Added to that was the time lost trying to find more expedient ways of getting there.

One particularly hot and stifling summer afternoon, on a day when the pavement seemed hot enough to melt, we warned the children to quickly roll up the rear car windows and make sure the door locks were down when we realized we were on a skidrow street littered with boozing derelicts. Their eyes popping with curiosity and fear, the children did as they were told. When, at last, we were able to locate a police car, we flagged it down to ask the uniformed driver how to get out of there fast. He shrugged, "Sorry, folks, I'm from out of town too, and I'm just as lost as you are!"

The winter trips through ice, wind, and snow were even more frightening. One night, coming back from an all-day clinic, we got caught in a blizzard during the Indiana stretch of the trip. The few motels we passed were either closed or full, and the weather conditions were much too dangerous to pull over to the side of the road. So for what seemed like endless hours, we tediously followed the red lights of a semitruck moving slowly ahead of us until we reached our own familiar exit. In the light of day, we wondered whether the truck driver had known that he had been our beacon leading us safely home.

Another cold, frosty night, returning home late from Shriners, Dick heard a noise under the hood and discovered the water pump was loose. "There aren't any garages open this time of night," he said. "We're going to have to risk making it home."

Holding our breaths, we drove through the frigid below-zero night until we were about ten miles from home. Then suddenly, a loud thump under the hood made Dick groan as he brought the car to a halt and jumped out to investigate the alarming sound.

"The water pump has let loose and pushed the fan into the radiator, and water is pouring out," he said as he reentered the car. "We're not going to make it home without water in the radiator to keep the car from heating up," he said.

I turned and looked at Mike sleeping soundly in his car bed in the backseat. "We can't just sit here waiting for help to come along. Not at this time of night. Not in this cold."

"No, we can't," Dick agreed. "There's a gas station not far from here. I'm sure it won't be open, but maybe we can make it that far and get some water or, at least, get to a phone."

The car clanked and chugged to the deserted gas station. But everything there was locked up tight, and the water that had been in an old can, sitting out by the gas pumps, was now a solid chunk of ice. "There's a creek close by. Maybe we can get some water there," Dick said hopefully.

Dully, I replied, "That'll be frozen too."

Grabbing a can and a screwdriver, Dick said, "Then I'll just have to break the ice."

Even though he must have known that pouring water into the damaged radiator would be of little or no help, he had to do something. Shivering with cold, he ran along the highway and down the bank to the frozen creek and came back a short while later, triumphantly holding a full can of water. The water didn't last long in the punctured radiator; it was barely enough to keep the car going. It's a wonder we didn't wake the entire neighborhood when finally we drove the clanging, smoking car into our driveway. Safe inside our warm, cozy house, Dick and I looked at each other as we both heaved a big sigh of relief. Exhausted from the long day at the clinic and the tension-filled ride home, I cried, "Why do we take these awful trips? We could have frozen to death out there!"

Looking in Mike's direction, Dick mouthed, "We do it for him."

There wasn't any cost-free overnight housing then, like there is today for families traveling to hospitals for specialized medical care for their children. Our tight budget precluded us from staying at elegant hotels like the one we had once picked by mistake, and that had nearly wiped out all our travel funds, as well as our food budget for the month. Nor did we want to repeat the night we had spent in a cheap motel, only to be kept awake throughout the night by the comings and goings of gentlemen callers to the room next door. The grunts, groans, and exclamations we had overheard through the thin walls had evoked way too many questions from Mike!

Most of the time, when he was scheduled for routine clinics, we rose very early, drove to Chicago, saw a doctor, then made the long trip back, often arriving home in the wee hours of the morning.

It was during one of the regular clinic visits that we met Dr. Edward Millar, the orthopedist replacing Dr. Sofield, who was retiring as chief surgeon. Calm and attentive was our initial assessment of the bespectacled, slightly balding man who was to have a very important role in our lives. From the start, Dr. Millar listened carefully to everything we had to say about Mike. He never brushed anything off as unimportant, never made us feel that we had no say in his treatment because we weren't paying for it.

Nearly two years after Mike's first hospitalization, Dr. Millar told us that Mike was outgrowing the rods in his legs and would have to be readmitted to have them replaced. Out of Mike's presence, he told us, "If everything goes well with the surgery, I'd like to get his legs into braces this time and try to get him up on his feet."

Amazement spread to both of our faces as the meaning of Dr. Millar's words sank in. Choking up, I asked, "Are you saying there's a possibility Mike could walk?"

Dr. Millar smiled patiently. "A possibility, yes, but a very remote one. First, we have to get him up on his feet. Only then will we be able to determine if he should try walking. It would mean a very long hospital stay—maybe as long as six or eight months."

The trip home that day was emotionally charged with an array of mixed feelings. One moment we were sad about Mike having to go away again for such a long time; the next, we bubbled with joy thinking about the remote chance that our child, who had once been doomed to live his life carried on a pillow like a china doll, might someday walk.

Not wanting to hurt or disappoint Mike if things didn't work out, we didn't tell him about the possibility of braces to help him stand up. All we said was that he was outgrowing his steel rods and would have to have them replaced. The length of time that he would have to be away from home was also kept from him. We knew that leaving again would be difficult enough without burdening him with a new list of hopeful expectations.

This time, however, Mike settled in at Shriners without much fuss. Sometimes, he even appeared to be happy to be back in the lively rooms with other children like him who had a disability and used some kind of conveyance on wheels to get around. Most of them used walkers, wheelchairs, or long carts on wheels nicknamed "banana" carts so they could recline with their cumbersome casts or other orthopedic appliances. Other than Mike and Peter Lollar, a boy from Arkansas, there were few patients in the wards with osteogenesis imperfecta. Because of this, Mike learned early on to use his fragility to his advantage. He also discovered that naughtiness resulted in time spent alone in the "quiet room."

Once, during his second stay, we arrived at the hospital after our long drive only to hear that we could see him for a limited visit since he was confined to the "quiet room" for instigating some mischief in the ward. This kind of punishment was harder on us than on him. But the surgery was going well, so we kept quiet about inconveniences like these.

Since Dr. Millar wasn't on duty when we visited on weekends, we saw a resident orthopedist who kept us informed of Mike's progress. Another Sunday afternoon, we learned that the surgical phase of Mike's hospital stay was over and that a physical therapist was exercising his legs daily in preparation for braces. Several weeks later, Mike beamed when he showed us the new braces that the resident explained were designed to put weight on his pelvis rather than on his legs.

"I've been practicing walking with a walker, then I'm going to try crutches," Mike confided when the resident had completed his rounds. The next visit, the walker and crutches were by his hospital bed, but he refused to show us how he was doing with them. He wasn't quite ready, he said, to try walking without the help of the therapist. Smiling smugly, he said, "Anyway, I want it to be a surprise when you come to take me home."

And what a wonderful surprise it was, that day of days that we could never have imagined. His tiny braces on and standing within the framework of the walker, his somewhat uncertain steps faltering a bit, Mike walked down the long hospital corridor to meet us. With Dr. Millar, the residents, and nurses cheering him on, he kept his bright, happy eyes focused on us until he reached our welcoming arms. It was a once-in-a-lifetime moment that we would never forget.

Chapter Eight

"We want Mike to go to St. Mary's School with Cathy. It's the perfect place for him," I remember telling the silver-haired pastor of our parish church.

Dick and I had helped with fund-raisers for the brand-new school with a ramped entrance that made the brightly painted classrooms wheelchair accessible.

Astonishment colored the priest's face red, and he blustered, "That's impossible, Mrs. Geisman. Our teachers aren't nurses. They're not trained to take care of sick children!"

"Mike's not sick!" I countered back. "He just has to be more careful because his bones break easily. He's very bright. He *needs* to be in school."

The pastor closed his eyes and folded his hands as if in prayer, as priests often do. Then looking at me with a semblance of sympathy, he said, "I'm sorry, we simply can't take the risk," and walked away.

"Father!" I called after him. "Can't he even come for religious instructions? You have ramps for his wheelchair. I'd stay with him the entire time he was here. We'd sign a paper releasing you of responsibility."

Turning to face me, he said, "I think it would be best if my assistant came to your house to give him his religious instructions."

Trembling and trying desperately not to cry, I flew out the door and drove home, furious at the pastor for blatantly disregarding the teachings of Jesus who had counseled his apostles to let the little children come unto him.

The public school system wouldn't take Mike either, but we were advised that, according to the law, he was entitled to five hours a week of home tutoring by an accredited teacher. Having no other choice, we agreed to take whatever was offered, which turned out to be four different teachers in less than two years. These were substitute teachers who loved Mike, entertained him, and spoiled him until a better position became available. Instead of teaching him how to read, they read to him. And rather than hurt his feelings, they didn't correct him when he held his pencil the wrong way. As a result of their pampering, Mike could barely read and write by the time Mrs. Williams came along.

You'd have thought that a wind gust had blown her in, the way she came breezing into our lives that warm March day, carrying a large satchel in one hand and a pile of books under her arm. Braced in the doorway, her fine-feathered hat perched jauntily on her head, she announced, "I'm Mrs. Williams. I'm here to teach Mike."

I called Mike away from the TV and introduced them. Without flinching, the way some of the other teachers had done when first confronted with Mike's physical condition, she reached for his hand and said, "Okay, Mike, let's get to work."

Appalled at the mention of work, Mike reluctantly followed behind us as I showed her to the study. After I had apologized for the rickety card table and the makeshift tray for Mike's wheelchair, she thanked me politely and shooed me out the door. "We'll get acquainted later," she said firmly. "Right now I have to teach Mike."

Uh-oh, I said to myself. *Mike has finally met his match. He's not going to con this teacher!*

Pulling Dickie up on my lap, we waited out that first long session quietly, rocking and listening to the steady hum of voices, punctuated with exclamation sounds from Mike, coming from behind the closed door. After what seemed like a very long time, the door flew open, and Mike called, "Mom! Dickie! Come here! Come see what I made!"

Dickie slipped off my lap when Mike appeared holding a brightly colored kite with a gingham tail sailing gaily behind it. My mouth dropped in disappointment. Was that what they had done? Was this teacher going to be like all the others who had entertained and spoiled Mike but had taught him little?

Seeing my reaction, she said, "Don't worry, Mother. We did our lessons first. The kite was made on *my* time."

"I've never had a kite before," Mike exclaimed, his eyes gleaming.

"A boy has to have some fun," Mrs. Williams confided with a wink of her merry eyes. "I promised him we'd make a kite if he worked hard. And he did. He worked very hard."

From that day on, that's the way it was. Mike learned steadily, and with each new task mastered, there was a bright reward. However, boys will be boys, and Mike was no exception. He knew all the tricks to get out of doing schoolwork, but he quickly discovered, to his dismay, that what had worked with her predecessors didn't work with the formidable Mrs. Williams.

Once, after she'd been with us for several weeks, she came stomping out of the study, looking harried but grimly determined. "Mother," she said evenly, "Mike has informed me that he won't study unless I go home early so he can watch the Tarzan movie on TV. He says—"

"Never mind what Mike says," I interrupted. "When you're here teaching, you're in charge."

Visibly relieved, she said, "I thought you felt that way, but I wanted to hear it from you." Giving me a glance of approval, she disappeared back into the study. This time, it was quite obvious that I had passed the teacher's test!

Despite her determination to ignore his demands, Mike tried to outwit her again and again, but the lady always had the upper hand.

As she was leaving one day, Mrs. Williams took me aside and whispered, "You want to hear the latest? Now he says that copying is against his religion."

"Copying?"

"Copying spelling words from his workbook for a homework assignment," she answered.

"That kind of copying is definitely not against our religion, but lying sure is," I said loud enough for Mike to hear.

Mike's face paled as hers crinkled up with laughter. "He thought he had me this time!" she said as she went out the door shaking her head.

Some people are born to teach. I knew almost right away that Bonnie Williams was one of them. She had the rare insight of knowing instinctively how to treat a child. She knew when to be tough, when to be gentle. She also knew that to get to know a child, you've got to know his family.

Whenever Cindy was home from kindergarten, she and Dickie would eagerly press their noses to the windowpane to watch for her. "Teacher's coming!" they'd announce to Mike when they spotted her little white car coming down the street.

The days she came were never dull. After the lessons were finished for the day, she'd enthrall all of us with stories about the places she'd lived, the sons she had reared, and the children she'd taught. There was an excitement for learning about her that soon became contagious.

There were times when I couldn't wait for Monday morning to come. There were so many things I wanted to discuss with her. I wanted her opinion when Krushchev was deposed and replaced by Brezhnev and Kosygin. I wondered what she thought about the frivolous Vietnamese Madame Ngo Dinh Nhu. Not that it mattered to anyone else, but it mattered to me that I finally had someone who was willing to discuss world affairs and current events instead of housekeeping and child-care topics. She respected my interest. Whenever I'd apologize for taking her time, she'd brush it off, saying, "Don't worry, taking part in our discussions is learning for Mike too."

It was learning for Mike, for all of us. Through her, worlds we had never known, that geography books couldn't teach, were revealed to us.

Once, when she left for a Florida trip, we felt as if we were going along. She had drawn the route of her trip on a map for us to follow her travels. When she returned, she had brought bits of Florida back to us. We held a sea horse and a starfish in our hands; we cupped seashells to our ears and heard distant ocean sounds. It was almost as if we were with her on a Florida beach with warm, wet sand clinging between our toes.

Another time, she shared vivid memories of a summer in the Minnesota woods with us. We sat in the sauna baths of an old Finnish farmhouse. We basked in the warmth of its fireplace. We saw deer nimbly prancing in the clearing and heard bears growling in the night. We went to so many places, saw so many things with her.

She brought enrichment in other ways too. In a matter-of-fact way, she gave Mike what every school student was entitled to and then some. In her large straw handbag, heaped with the wonderful world of books, came stories about famous men who had overcome handicaps. George Washington Carver, the Negro boy who overcame poverty and hardship to become a famous scientist, so inspired Mike that he tried to find out for himself how many ways he could use peanut butter. He thrilled to the heroism of John F. Kennedy when on PT 109 and was excited to discover that Johnny Appleseed had scattered seeds right in our own Midwest area, maybe even across the street from us where an apple orchard stood!

She brought him books about the weather, space, the world until he was aware and interested in every aspect of the big world outside his own small sphere. She also brought him fun books, the kind that brought laughter into a little boy's otherwise uneventful life.

What he couldn't go to, she brought to him. Valentine's Day, Easter, Thanksgiving—all were celebrated with social flare. "He has to have those things," she insisted. "They're part of learning too!"

I'll never forget the Christmas that she brought the holiday spirit to us in a big brown paper bag. She appeared at the door that day, her cheeks red and looking like Mrs. Santa Claus. I didn't know what she was up to, but after months of knowing her, I knew that whatever it was, it was special. With a twinkle in her eyes, she closed the study door. It was obvious that her plans were for an intimate gathering of two.

I gasped at the transformation that had taken place in the study when the children and I were later invited in. It seemed an altogether different room. The old card table had been turned into an elegant buffet, beautifully adorned with a paper tablecloth and lighted candles of old-fashioned brown wax circled with holly leaves. Christmas goodies were heaped high on paper plates, and there were dainty holiday napkins and cups filled with sparkling ginger ale for each one of us. I don't think I had ever seen Mike enjoy Christmas as much as he was enjoying it that day with her.

Bonnie Williams taught Mike for almost three years. But one bright sunny day in June, when school was ending, we all knew she wasn't coming back. Mike was scheduled to go away for months of surgery at Shriners, and she had accepted a post in the new remedial-reading program in our community.

"I've opened the doors for Mike," she said as she was preparing to leave on her last day. "I hope I haven't been too hard on him."

"Too hard!" I cried in disbelief. "You were the perfect teacher for him. You were the medicine he needed. You not only opened the doors, you led him into new worlds!"

Tears welled in her eyes. "There's one thing I couldn't give him," she said, "and that's the companionship of schoolmates and the competition of the classroom. I hope he'll have both someday."

Mike turned his head to hide away his tears when she left. I think he would have traded a hundred Tarzan movies for her to stay.

As for her, she simply put on her teacher's face and sternly said, "Now, Mike, you work hard, you hear?" And she was gone. Gone the same as she had arrived, without much fanfare, and acting as if the gift of learning that she had brought to all of us was just part of her job.

That was her way. But I knew, as I watched her walk away, that none of us would ever forget the woman who had come to teach, but had given us so much more.

Chapter Nine

Mike's ability to walk didn't last. In spite of our faithful daily routine of leg and arm exercises and time spent tediously walking with crutches around our large kitchen, he regressed. At first, when the walking had been new, I had hovered behind him, ready to grab his T-shirt if he began to wobble or fall. He had laughed. "Mom, let me go! I can do it!" With much reluctance, I had buried my fears and let him go.

Now, every morning when it was time to walk, he went into a panic. "Mom, hold on to me. Don't let me fall!" Or "I don't want to walk anymore. My legs hurt! I want my wheelchair!"

Dick and I were worried. We had noticed small bumps below the surgical scars on Mike's legs and wondered whether they were the cause of his pain and discomfort when walking. Sounding horrified, Dick called me into the bathroom one day while he was giving Mike a bath. "I know what the bumps are," he said. "They're his rods working their way out of the bone and coming through his skin."

I looked at the protrusions on Mike's legs and could almost see the tips of the rods through his translucent skin. Swallowing hard not to get sick, I fled from the bathroom. A few days later, one of the lumps appeared red and infected, so we phoned Shriners and spoke to a resident. As if it was an everyday occurrence, and it probably was to him, he said, "The rod needs to come out, but there's no need for you to come all the way to Chicago. If it's that close to the surface, you probably can pull it out yourselves. It's as simple as pulling a loose tooth." My loud gasp on the telephone line must've alerted him to suggest a more sensible alternative. "Or," he hurried to add, "you can take him to your hospital's emergency room."

The medical personnel at the emergency room were also very reluctant to do it. They knew that because of Mike's fragility, they could very well fracture his leg while attempting to pull out the rod. We had to promise to absolve them of any liability before they would proceed. We did, and as Dick and I stood helplessly by, they pulled the rod out to the sound of Mike's bloodcurdling screams.

A feeling of devastation followed us home from the emergency room. In the bottom of my purse was the small stainless steel rod that had signified so much hope. In my heart was a feeling of desolation like I had never known before. It was as if we had just been witness to the death of hope.

The entire country was going through a similar period of desolation. John F. Kennedy had been murdered at the hands of an assassin. Bobby Kennedy and Martin Luther King had suffered the same fate. Riots and burnings were destroying our cities, and a senseless war was raging in Vietnam, the land that my missionary brother had been forced to flee after more than twenty years of ministering to the Vietnamese.

For a while now, I too had been festering with feelings of disillusionment. At that point in my life, I seldom heard from the scattered members of my large family other than an occasional letter from my aging mother and two of my sisters, Gerry and Fernande. They were all very busy rearing their own children. Mrs. Williams, who had been a bright presence in my life, was gone. Dick was working night and day trying to establish a new cleaning business, and his mother had remarried. Cathy was spending more and more time with her own friends, and Cindy and her cousin Christy had become inseparable. Weekends, we often spent time with Dick's brother Jim and his wife, Mary; but weekdays, when school was not in session, it was usually Mike, Dickie, and I. When school was in session, it was Mike and I and an occasional teacher. Other mothers had jobs, were developing careers, were seeing people and socializing. So why was it that *I* had been singled out for a life of senseless confinement in a prison of impossible dreams?

Having the rod pulled out of Mike's leg seemed to have triggered even more ambivalence. The stares of people, the finger-pointing, the rude questions from strangers—"What's the matter with him? Oh dear, what's wrong with his arms and legs? Why is his head so big? Why is it flat in the back? Is he retarded?"—made me want to scream. A Pandora's box of feelings was opening and releasing all that I had smothered for so long.

At first, I blamed myself for Mike's failure to walk, to thrive, and to grow normally. After a while, without consciously realizing it, I began blaming him. More and more, I was turning away from his loving gestures. And I was expressing my unhappiness by constantly complaining about the tasks I had to do to keep him clean and fed. Eventually, I found myself thinking about how much easier life was when Mike was away, how much freer I was.

An untamed shrew had taken residence inside me, tormenting me, taunting, pulling me in every direction. To banish those thoughts and feelings, I'd often tell myself, *I love Mike. It's* osteogenesis imperfecta *I hate!*

In a sense, I had faced the fact that Mike would never be normal or able to walk the way other children did. I knew all the facts, but I had not fully accepted them. Over time, the dreams and the hoping had turned into a frightening nightmare.

On a hot summer day, when everything had seemed to go wrong, I finally reached the breaking point. I had gone upstairs to get Mike after his afternoon nap. As usual, I grumbled as I picked him up to carry him downstairs. I hadn't gone far when something made me stop.

Do it now! Get it over with! the shrew inside me coaxed. *You could say it was an accident, that you tripped!*

I trembled. It was so hot, I could hardly breathe. My arms relaxed around their burden, my hands loosened.

Then for a brief moment, my eyes met Mike's eyes, filled with love and trust; and my own love for him reacted, and instinctively, my arms formed a tight, protective circle around him. "Don't hold me so tight, Mommy!" he squealed. "You're squashing me!"

I wanted to hold him even tighter, never to let him go. But giving in to his plea, I carried him down the rest of the stairs and gently placed him into his waiting wheelchair.

When he had wheeled himself away, I went to my room and wept. I needed to thank God for letting me know during that brief moment just how much I loved my son. It was clear to me now that I had pretended to hate because it had hurt too much to love.

Not everything was perfect after that eye-opening experience. Now more than ever, I wanted life to be better for Mike—for all of us. So when my missionary brother, Irenee, who was now rector at the Basilica of St. Anne de Beaupre in the Province of Quebec in Canada, invited us to come visit the shrine where miraculous cures had been documented, we jumped at another chance to ask for a miracle for Mike.

For weeks, we planned our trip. But shortly, before we were to leave, we received a letter from Shriners Hospital informing us that Mike was scheduled to be admitted to have his rods replaced the week of our planned pilgrimage to St. Anne's.

Rereading the letter, I cried, "How can we go to St. Anne's without Mike! It's for him that we're going!"

Appearing as crestfallen as I was, Dick too read the letter again. "I guess God has other plans for Mike," he said dejectedly.

"Well, if he can't go, then none of us will!" I said. I turned as I spoke, and there was Mike beside me, his lower lip quivering.

"Mom, you go to St. Anne's without me," he said. "I know you've always wanted to go."

Stubbornly, I replied, "No, we're not going without you!"

He objected, "But, Mom, you're the one who wants a miracle, please go."

I looked at him and thought, *Dear God, doesn't he realize we're doing this for him?* Out loud, I gave in. "All right. We'll go. I guess I'll have to do the asking for you."

We left for St. Anne's several days after Mike had been readmitted to Shriners. It didn't seem right to be going without him, but I was determined to beg his cause.

The beauty and majesty of the hillside, the village, the Basilica of St. Anne left us breathless with wonder. Like the other pilgrims, we toured the grounds, attended the evening mass and the candlelight procession. During the ceremony, I glanced at Dick, and his eyes moistened as he looked at the invalids in their wheelchairs. "I wish Mike was here," he whispered.

We saw and enjoyed the physical wonders of St. Anne's: the wax museum that depicted the life of the grandmother of Jesus, the ornate altars, and the hillside Way of the Cross. We climbed the Holy Stairs on our knees, and when we were done, I remember telling my brother, "Darn, my knees hurt!"

Irenee looked at me, smiled his serene smile, and replied, "They're *supposed* to hurt."

On our last day at St. Anne's, we got up early and attended a special mass said in Mike's behalf by my brother. As I knelt with my family, I thought, *Well, no miracle yet!* Then as I continued to pray, it gradually became clear to me that my appeals for a miracle for Mike lacked a certain candor and sincerity, even to my own ears. Thinking back to what Mike had said to me when we had learned that he'd be unable to come with us, I realized that *he* had known all along that I was the one who had needed to come to St. Anne's, that the miracle I had been praying for had not been for him, but for me!

With new awareness, I resumed my prayers. This time, I didn't ask for a miracle. Instead, I asked for stronger love, more patience, a better understanding of Mike's disability, and whatever other help I would need to become a better mother to all my children. It hurt to think about all I had put my family through while I'd searched for a miracle for Mike when all the while, the greatest need had been mine. It hurt. But hadn't my brother just told me that some things were *supposed* to hurt?

Part Two

There is in every true woman's heart a spark of heavenly fire, which lies dormant in the broad daylight of prosperity; but which kindles up, and beams and blazes in the dark hour of adversity.
　　　　—Washington Irving, *The Sketch Book* (1819-1820)

Chapter Ten

Parting with secret thoughts that have been sheltered for a long time is like having an abscessed tooth pulled. It hurts.

Anticipating the pain, I had anesthetized myself with large doses of confidence during the months that preceded publication of my story in *Redbook. The feelings we'd had about OI were for sharing*, I told myself. Perhaps they'd help others to understand that ambivalence can and often does exist in the hearts of those who are caregivers of the sick or disabled.

How flimsy my protection was! Only hours after the magazine hit the newsstands nationwide, my assurance had completely dissipated. The mother of another sick child was the first to inform me that I was wicked to have written what I had, that a good and decent mother would never harbor the feelings I'd described. She said *she* thanked God every single day for giving *her* a "special" child. Soon after that encounter, I discovered that she wasn't the only one who felt that way.

Acquaintances, friends, even people I had thought sympathetic, avoided me. The more daring scrutinized me with bold, condemning looks. To be scorned and denounced so openly for telling my story honestly was a disheartening turn that I had not entirely expected.

My mother had always claimed an extrasensory perception when it came to her children. We had laughed and told her that what she had wasn't ESP, but motherly intuition multiplied by thirteen. Whatever it was, it didn't fail her when I needed her. Seventy-five years old and recovering from cataract surgery, still speaking in her native French Canadian dialect and barely able to read English, she attempted to read my story written in words she scarcely understood. Then with characteristic simplicity, she wrote me a note that, in essence, said, "I'm so very proud of you for speaking out. Keep your spirits up. God will reward you someday."

She didn't mention the heartaches and suffering. Nor did she say that she'd had similar feelings while raising her large brood. Yet it was quite clear to me that she understood my pain. It may have been sheer coincidence, but after Ma's simple note, the tide of negative responses began to turn.

From her convent far away, my spiritual counselor since childhood, my eldest sister, Fernande, wrote the following:

My precious little sister,

Through the years we have always communed well with one another, haven't we? We are much the same. Sometimes I even think of you as my "alter ego," my other self, and I have always thought I understood you like no one else. As I read your poignant story, I tried as a woman to put myself in your place so I could understand your feelings. I can honestly say that I know how you felt. I understand. You were brave and courageous to put it all down on paper. Had it been me, I don't think I could have done it. I love you now more than ever. You are and always will be my special gem, and I'm proud that I had something to do, however small, in the cutting and polishing of that precious stone.

Healing words. Welcomed. Embraced. Others followed, but it was this, along with Ma's, that set off a chain reaction of positive responses from the rest of the family and the world.

For several weeks, I had been castigated. Now, because of the appearance of sympathetic newspaper stories, I was being declared a courageous mother, a wonderful woman, even a saint! Church groups approached me to speak at their meetings, but still hurting, I refused. Though I wanted, more than anything, to have them understand the problems associated with raising a child born with a rare, incurable disorder, I still did not have the courage to address the difficulties and realities in that particular setting. I needed more time to sort out and learn how to cope with the diverse reactions to my story and to figure out how I would answer the questions that no doubt would arise during live presentations. I wasn't yet aware that I had awakened an urgent desire in others who needed to talk about their own secret anguish.

I began to learn this when an eighty-year-old man, a friend of the family, phoned me to reveal that he had never told anyone that he'd placed a mentally retarded son in an institution many years before. "All these years!" he sobbed as he tried to explain why he and his wife had done it.

"You don't have to explain anything to me," I told him, but he begged to be heard.

"I want you to know what it means to me to be able to talk to someone about it," he said. "I've kept this a secret for so many years. What a heavy burden it's been. Now my wife's gone, and I'm too old to carry it alone any longer. I wanted you to know that I've had feelings like yours, and I've been so ashamed . . . so ashamed." His voice quivered, drifted off, and stopped. After he'd regained his composure somewhat, he continued, "All this time, I thought there was something terribly wrong, terribly monstrous about me. All these years . . ." Again, he began to sob, and this time, too shaken to continue, he hung up. I should have been drenched in his misery, but instead, I felt a comforting peace as I realized that my being there to listen had helped ease years of despair and guilt feelings for him.

Another acquaintance, a mother, told me that she too had a mentally ill son tucked away in an institution. I was amazed that I hadn't known since we had worked together on church and community projects. Now, having read my story, she felt comfortable revealing the feelings of frustration and hopelessness she'd had when she'd had to face the certainty that nothing could be done to bring her child out of his remote existence. Giving him up to the care of an institution had been their only choice, she confessed, if they were to preserve their own sanity and the well-being of their other children. As she spoke, I got the impression that she envied me my physically disabled son. "He's with you. He knows you're his mother. That's something mine will never know," she said with a hopelessness that far exceeded mine.

"After we read your article, my husband and I were able to talk to each other openly for the first time since our Mongoloid child was born," a young mother told me over the phone. "For years, we've pretended that the problem didn't exist because we were too afraid to face it. Like you, we thought that if we didn't look at it, it would go away! If you only knew how many times I've been tempted to put a pillow over his little face to end the misery and the nightmare! There were days when I thought all sanity had left me. I was so disgusted with myself, I wanted to die. Thank heavens your story came when it did. You may have saved my life and that of my child."

The confidences of others rest heavily in the heart of the listener. I had thought that revealing my emotions publicly would rid me of them. Instead, the load had become heavier and more complex. At times, it felt good to be able to help others with their problems, but most of the time, during those climactic weeks that followed publication, I yearned for the quiet, hopeful days that had preceded it.

Then one by one, the brash and bossy, supportive and loving, well-meant, funny fan letters began to arrive. Some offered sure-fire cures for Mike. Or elaborate diets were sent by amateur nutritionists who were convinced that well-balanced meals were the answer to his bone condition. Others exhorted the value of certain vitamin combinations. Professional miracle workers were recommended, and our names were added to the prayer lists of many religious denominations. Most of those who took the time to write did so to send their own personal messages of hope and understanding. All the letters were read and answered and reread again.

For instance, the very first letter I received from the public at large came from a woman who couldn't relate with my experiences since we had little in common. Yet in her letter was a genuine understanding of the message of love that I'd hoped to convey in my article.

The letter arrived on a cold, blustery February day, wrongly addressed and passed on to me by a neighbor who had discovered it in her mailbox. As I opened it, I marveled that it had found me at all. Expecting the condemning words I was becoming accustomed to, I sat down and read the following:

Dear Mrs. Geisman:

I have just finished reading your story in the March issue of *Redbook* and would like to thank you from the bottom of my heart for sharing your true feelings with me. I cannot say that I too have shared your experiences, for I haven't. I am the oldest of nine children. They are all healthy, beautiful and well-adjusted. I'm twenty-six years old and have remained single because I'm not sure I could be the person you have proved to be.

Your "four" children are beautiful and I thank God for giving us the ones just a little bit different to teach mankind the true meaning of the word *love*. God bless you all your days.

The wind howled outdoors. Snow and sleet hit against the windowpane, and a cold, penetrating draft filtered in beneath the door. But all I felt was this stranger's warmth and sincere words.

"The Lord thy God in the midst of thee is mighty" was the inscription on the cheery notepaper that brought me a message from a teacher in Michigan.

"Your story made me want to write to you," she said. "It will be very helpful to me in counseling parents, although the children I teach are not handicapped in the same way Mike is. The children in my primary room are educable, mentally handicapped ones between the ages of seven and twelve. I love each one of them and find working with them challenging and rewarding. Please don't think for a minute that we teachers never get discouraged or impatient. We certainly do, although the other times when we're thrilled and delighted far overshadow them."

Another letter, from a woman with OI, brought me my first hope that Mike might someday become an independent adult. She wrote the following:

Dear Mrs. Geisman,

I have thought of you often since reading your article. I am older than you, but I am still a small person like your son Mike. I smiled to read that he is the master organizer of the neighborhood gang. I did that too. "We" built playhouses and miniature golf courses! I feel it helped me develop a taste for independence.

My sister, who is younger than me, has given me a good life by including me in hers. I went through grade school with her, my parents taking me in a stroller-type buggy in the morning and rushing me home at noon for lunch. I often went half-days only but kept up my lessons at home. There were no tutors then, and I couldn't go to high school because of the stairs.

I've had my own apartment for six years now. To become independent was a long, slow process. I was in fourth grade before I learned to sit up from a lying down position.

I was over twenty before I realized I could slide down from the sofa into my walker. Then, when I was sure the walker wouldn't tip, I reversed the procedure and lifted myself up. Oh, how independent I felt then!

You're doing fine with Mike. If there is any way I can encourage or help, please let me know.

Other stories, similar to that one, followed. Another OI woman told me that she went to work as a receptionist, doing much of her daily tasks from the seat of a little red tricycle. A New York housewife with OI told me about her job, her new home, and her wheelchair-bound husband. Only three feet tall and deformed by frequent fractures, she appeared to have a happy life and marriage.

A Massachusetts woman with OI wrote that she was married and the mother of a normal seventeen-year-old boy. "At this point in my life, osteogenesis imperfecta has become a gift instead of a cross," she wrote. "With the help of God, Mike is on his way to a happy life because he is secure in your love. You and your family have been chosen for something special. Maybe you don't think so now. But wait, someday you will know it has all been worth it!"

Hers were prophetic words that wouldn't be understood by me for many more years. At that particular moment in time, I could not foresee ever thinking of OI as a gift.

However, to say that I wasn't amazed and encouraged by these letters would be untrue. For so long, we'd been told that Mike could never hope to live a normal and independent adult life. Now these letters were telling us that it *was* possible. Sharing some of these letters with Mike gave a big boost to his self-confidence. So much so that he began talking about becoming a Major League Baseball team manager or, someday, even president of the United States!

Every day when I gathered the fan letters from the mailbox, I hoped there would be one from another mother with an OI child—one who could fully empathize with my experiences.

At last, such a letter did arrive. The envelope, posted airmail, was marked Urgent. Pulling out several sheets of yellow-lined paper, I read the following:

Dear Gemma,

I don't know if you'll ever receive this letter. I hope you will because I want you to know that we too have an eleven-year-old son who has osteogenesis imperfecta.

I have just finished reading your story in *Redbook* magazine, and as I think back, I understand your story more than I can say.

Our son was born with only two fractures. It was such an easy delivery, he didn't break any more at birth. However, we were in a military hospital, and no one would tell me what was wrong with him. My husband had to leave right after the baby's birth, so I was alone and too young and too scared to find out more.

Finally, a teacher of mine got the Red Cross to help me reach a doctor who would talk to me about my baby. He told me what was wrong with him then told me to take him home because there was nothing he could do for him. At six weeks, I took him home.

Remember how terrible it was just to change a diaper? Every time they'd cry, you'd wonder if you had broken an arm or leg?

Now, my husband, Wayne, is in Vietnam, and tomorrow, I must take our son to the hospital for surgery. It's the first time I've had to face this alone. I haven't told Wayne because it worries him so much. It's better to tell him afterwards. Our boy always has such a bad reaction to the anesthetic, it worries us more than the actual surgery.

I often wonder if it's worth putting him through all the pain and suffering. Like you, I know that my son will probably never walk. He's in a wheelchair now and goes to public school and gets along well in spite of everything.

We have four other children younger than Cameron, all normal and healthy. Don't you find that the other children help a lot by accepting the handicapped one so well?

Oh, I hope you get this! Because now I have a slight hope for a cure for our boys. A doctor, a biochemist in Denver, has been experimenting by giving magnesium oxide to Cam and another OI child. We have only just started with him, but I feel he may be on to something worthwhile. He has been working with a child from Longmont, Colorado, for some time now and the child is definitely improving. No one knows why. Only that he was born with forty or more fractures and, now, at the age of four, is walking. Of course, his mother works with him for hours every day, exercising. You wouldn't believe what she has done for him!

If you would like to know more about this doctor, I can send you his name and address. I'm sure he'd be interested in hearing from you. In any case, it was wonderful reading your story. I'm especially happy that you've come to love your son so much. I too can remember hollering at Cam because I had to do things for him, still do I guess. But he has taught us so much—patience, love we could never have known without him. I've seen him suffer so much, I've often wondered why God didn't take him. Yet if something happened to him, I'd want to die! He's such a wonderful, happy little boy.

Write to me, if you can. I want to hear all about you and your family.

Sincerely,
Beverly

As soon as I finished Beverly's letter, I responded. I didn't want to lose the sense of sharing her letter had brought. Besides, I was very anxious to find out more about the doctor she had mentioned.

A few days later, another airmail letter from Beverly arrived with the doctor's name and address and a whole lot more motherly exchanges.

Beverly and I corresponded for a short while before she had a long siege of illness and had to be hospitalized. When Cam had to have further surgery, complications followed, and Wayne had to be brought back from Vietnam to help care for their family.

However, I remain forever grateful to Beverly for taking the time to write to me when things were so difficult for her. Had it not been for her, I may never have heard about the doctor from Denver and the mother and child from Longmont.

Chapter Eleven

Put in touch with one another by Beverly, Becky Keller and I began to correspond. From her very first letter, Becky's story began to unfold.

On April 22, 1964, her son, Doug, had been delivered breech and found to have somewhere between thirty-five to forty fractures. Twelve hours later, he had been diagnosed with a severe case of osteogenesis imperfecta congenita with no hope given for his survival. Six days later, after having undergone surgery for a groin hernia, the infant had been dismissed from the hospital with a warning to the parents that any exertion, even a sneeze, could be fatal. At seven weeks, he underwent further surgery for a groin hernia on the opposite side.

By the time he was two months old, Doug had already passed his predicted life expectancy and had encountered more pain and surgery than the average person experiences in a lifetime. Yet amazingly, it wasn't until a month later that the full impact of their child's illness hit Becky and Charles.

It was summer and deathly hot—a dry, searing, dehydrating heat, desertlike as only it can get hot in Colorado. Becky and Charles, dressed casually in their usual Western-style clothes, had driven to Denver from Cactus Patch Ranch, situated thirty-five miles north, to keep an appointment made for them by their pediatrician. It had been his suggestion that they obtain genetic counseling there.

Both raised in the Longmont area, the Kellers were used to the beauty of the mountains and the feel of the land. Denver, with its hustle and bustle, was usually avoided.

As they approached the sprawling complex of the medical center and walked up to the tall, towering building, Becky clutched the small bundle she carried close to her breast to quiet the pounding terror in her heart. Quietly supporting the arm that held the child, Charles led them into the vast lobby and approached the battery of desks to ask for assistance in locating the room number they'd been given. A smiling volunteer led them to a bank of elevators, then up several floors, down endless corridors, through numerous doors, and finally into a small cool waiting room. There, they were instructed to fill out forms. When that was completed, they were ushered into an examining room and asked to undress the baby so he could be weighed and measured.

This done, Becky and Charles sat silently with Doug, each wondering what would come next. They didn't have long to speculate. Suddenly, a group of medical men swarmed into the room, introduced themselves, and immediately began to ask questions and record answers.

"After what seemed like hours of questioning, we were joined by two other doctors who attempted to examine Doug without touching him," Becky wrote. "I think it was then that I fully realized just how fragile my baby was. I was asked to turn him, hold him upright, lay him down, and turn him onto his stomach. At no time did anyone attempt to handle him or move his arms or legs. These big strong men, who had seen all sorts of crippling diseases, seemed gripped with a fear of hurting him, and that frightened me too."

As suddenly as they had appeared, the doctors waltzed out of the room to confer. "The sudden aloneness after the barrage of questions turned to near hysteria. *What are they saying?* we wondered out loud. *What did we tell them? What will they tell us?* Oh, the things that went through our minds as we waited in that room! We sensed that some sort of sentence was being deliberated, that our baby's future and ours was in the hands of the doctors who had interrogated us. Waiting for the verdict was unbearable.

"We had a right to be concerned. When they returned, the initial prognosis had not changed. Only this time, it seemed more real, more final. They tried to be kind when they told us that Doug would probably not live long. And if by some miracle he did survive, he would never walk, sit, or hold his head up unaided. The bone disorder was a hereditary defect of genetic origin, they said, and they advised us not to have any other children. Aside from Doug, we have another son, Joe, who was nine years old at the time and perfectly healthy. We were told to be grateful and consider him and Doug our family."

Outdoors again, the sun shone brilliantly. Becky blinked at the sudden brightness and shivered. A cold numbness that even the hot Colorado sun couldn't thaw permeated her being. Her head ached, and the perspiring baby felt like a small wet bird in her arms. Charles appeared drawn and extremely tired as he guided them both to the car. At that moment, the uncomplicated life they'd had at Cactus Patch Ranch seemed to have been swallowed up into the vast unknown that was osteogenesis imperfecta.

They were strangely silent as they rode. So many words had been spoken. What did they all mean? How would they affect the rest of their lives? If Doug lived, he would never walk, sit, or even hold his head up unassisted. They'd have to plan a future with a child who would be bedridden and would need constant care—a child who wouldn't grow like other children. Was that what they had been told? Surely not! It couldn't be true!

Days passed—days filled with agony, grief, and bitter tears. A deep depression engulfed Becky, and she, in turn, engulfed those around her. It was a difficult time for everyone, and Becky was reluctant to remember any of it, yet now she now felt the need to share it with me.

"What finally drew us up and out of our deep sorrow is hard to say. I think it was a combination of people and things rather than one particular event. First of all, a wonderful public health nurse with a lifetime of wisdom on which to draw came to our rescue. She spent hours helping and talking to us, discussing bone problems in general. She encouraged mild forms of exercise and fresh air. She told us to keep Doug away from visitors with colds and flu since respiratory diseases were the chief causes of death in babies with OI. In short, she advised plain common sense care. Just talking with someone who understood was a beginning. Second, was a family that encouraged me to do my best and tried to give me the courage to do what I thought was right. The next, and perhaps the thing that really saw me through, is an inborn streak of stubbornness that, to this day, makes me mad at the gloomy predictions that are always associated with OI. You are all wrong, I wanted to shout. My baby will live. He will too hold his head up and sit!"

The attractive tall brunette had a fighting spirit that would not allow her to wallow in misery and despair for long. Gradually, she began to accept the challenge of caring for her newborn son. It was a slow, tedious learning process, but eventually, ideas to help Doug were tried. Some were quickly discarded as too dangerous; others were adopted as safe and useful. I could almost hear Becky chuckle between the lines as she remembered some of the earlier experiments. These were the good memories that she loved to share.

"We dug out a big old-fashioned bathtub, the kind people used to drag into the middle of the floor on Saturday nights. We fitted it with a spigot. A table was arranged with huge casters, and the tub mounted on the table. Three times a day, I wheeled the whole mess into the bathroom and filled the tub with warm water and began my own ideas of how to help Doug learn to move without breaking to pieces. We played and splashed like two idiots! Anything I could devise to make him kick and move in the water was not overlooked. Eventually, it paid off. After about three months of these daily workouts, Doug held his head erect and peeked cautiously over my shoulder."

With a lot of hard work, Becky and Charles had battled one of the odds and won. Doug was holding his head up unaided. If he could do that, then he could learn to sit and walk. Month followed month. Doug could sit on his mother's lap, but not alone. Then one day, he rolled over by himself, and everyone was overjoyed that it had happened without a fracture. Small triumphs like these were eagerly divulged during visits to their pediatrician. His responses were encouraging, but still cautious.

At the end of one such visit, the doctor casually mentioned to the Kellers that he had heard that a man from South Africa was due to arrive in Denver soon to start work on some research projects into birth defects, particularly into bone abnormalities. This gave Becky hope. Without hesitating, she told the pediatrician that when the man arrived, she wanted to be first in line to see him. He agreed to arrange it.

"Charles and I were so eager to do everything we could to help Doug that we recklessly defaced the house or anything else we owned if we thought it would be useful to encourage our tiny boy to move at all. Balloons were hung on walls with thumbtacks to encourage him to kick at them with his spindly legs. Soft balls were purchased and abandoned in favor of balloons for games of catch. Balls of yarn dangled from ceilings. Sometimes, I even held Doug in a sitting position on top of the automatic washer and encouraged him to play drums on the washer with his heels. Any silly game to make him use his limbs."

Aside from the therapeutic games, Doug loved the animals about the ranch best. His favorite pastime was romping with the cats and dogs in the household. His next favorite was doing chores with Dad or big brother, Joe. He had no inkling whatsoever that he was different in any way from other kids.

Between the triumphs and the fun, there were some nightmare trips to the doctor when Doug cried in acute pain. The parents of a baby with OI don't know, most of the time, whether the baby has a fracture or is crying from colic or other discomforts. There is always the ever-present fear of fractures, and Becky and Charles were not spared. Each time Doug cried excessively, or seemed to hurt, they had him examined and x-rayed. And each time a fracture was not detected, they breathed a sigh of relief.

During one of these visits to the pediatrician, they heard that the research doctor from South Africa was due to arrive soon. More time passed. More homegrown experiments were tried, more exercises, more visits to the doctor. Then finally, the awaited news—the researcher had arrived! An appointment followed, then came another wait.

This interval exacted new questions. Who was this man? Would his experiments hurt? Would they jeopardize the progress Doug was making? Did he know anything at all about osteogenesis imperfecta ? Would he understand the problems associated with it? So few did. Would Doug matter to him as a person, or would he view him as some kind of guinea pig?

Finally, the day to find the answers out arrived. For the second time since Doug's birth, Becky entered the mammoth medical center with a mixture of fear and hope. Again, she was led to the elevators, down wide corridors, through a door marked Pediatrics, down another hallway, flanked by many doors, each marked with the name of some research project or other. Suddenly, one of the doors popped open, and a man with a friendly and brightly smiling face held out a greeting hand. "You must be Mrs. Keller," he said. "I'm Dr. Solomons. Please come in."

Meeting Dr. Solomons was a huge step forward for the Kellers. It wasn't that he knew so much more about OI. His eagerness to work with them, to find out all he could about it was what appealed to them.

They talked about many things that first day. Becky spoke about her successes with Doug. The doctor, in turn, told her about his education, his research background as a biochemist, and about his particular interest in childhood diseases for which there was no known cure. Future appointments were arranged, and Becky left for home feeling a flickering gleam of hope for Doug and other children like him.

From then on, each small feat accomplished by Doug was reported to Dr. Solomons, who urged them to keep trying. "We're getting somewhere," he'd say. And indeed, they were. On his first birthday, Doug sat alone in his high chair to blow out his single candle.

"The next year brought a multitude of appointments with Dr. Solomons. We became quite fond of him. He was always so kind, so enthusiastic, and he seemed to love Doug as much as we did. We talked with him, sometimes for hours, and much of ourselves was bared to him. Our feeling was that the more he knew about us, the better he could help Doug. There were many interviews and discussions. Dr. Solomons was curious about every aspect of living with Doug and was also vitally interested in anything we could reveal about our child and his condition. We laughingly referred to his curiosity as 'brain picking.'

"That summer was spent trying to record everything Doug ate with the hope that some information could be gained from it. However, by that time, Doug was sitting alone on the floor, and I'm sure I missed some dirt, bugs, and other assorted things on those charts!"

During their many conversations with Dr. Solomons, Becky mentioned that Doug suffered greatly from the heat and often perspired profusely. This small fact appeared very interesting to Dr. Solomons. He ordered the menu charts continued and requested collections of twenty-four-hour urine output for five consecutive days for study. This was done, then more visits followed, more questions, more discussions. The work was time-consuming and very slow. Sometimes, even after weeks of probing and testing, nothing had been gained. "But," Becky told me, "suddenly, one morning, I realized that I was not dreading the visits to the medical center any longer, nor was I fearing the great big doors swinging shut behind me as I had before. It was late summer and very hot and miserable, and I was walking through those doors with anticipation rather than dread. Dr. Solomons, with his enthusiasm to learn, had done that for me."

After his concentrated study of the urine specimens, Dr. Solomons decided to try Doug on medication—a fine white powder known as magnesium oxide. It was experimental, on two weeks, off two weeks, then on again. Everyone watched with anticipation for outward signs of change, but none were immediately apparent. No one could visibly see what was happening, but the urine specimens seemed to be telling Dr. Solomons something. So he ordered blood tests. Maybe he was on to something.

The Kellers grew excited. That is, all the Kellers except Doug. Like any small child, Doug hated the testing and probing, and he took to crying and screaming whenever he saw anyone dressed in white.

Nevertheless, the tests continued over his frantic objections. The entire family, including any and all relatives willing to be tested, participated. Some drove distances, others flew—anything to help Dr. Solomons find a way to help Doug.

The major drawback for the ongoing project was the fact that Dr. Solomons had only Doug to work with. One case would not prove anything, and the scarcity of patients to study disturbed the doctor. To help him, Becky began to search for others with OI. She wrote to a woman in Pennsylvania, who reputedly kept a national registry of people with OI. She sent requests to a Texas OI Foundation, but her letters came back unopened. Doctors and hospitals were contacted, again without success. If she saw or heard news stories about anyone who might remotely be connected in any way with OI, she wrote, but hardly ever got a response.

Then one day, a friend who knew about her search phoned her. "Becky, I just heard a plea on the radio for cards for a little boy with OI who is a patient at Fitzsimmons Hospital. I thought you'd like to know."

Becky sent a card and note and, by return mail, received a long letter from Beverly, who was living in nearby Thornton while her husband, Wayne, was serving in Vietnam. Telephone calls followed. Both mothers talked endlessly about their sons and made arrangements to meet to compare experiences.

During a visit at Cactus Patch Ranch, and while their children played nearby, Becky told Beverly about Dr. Solomons's research and about his desperate need for more patients to study. Within a week, the two mothers were meeting in North Denver and driving to the medical center together.

Dr. Solomons found the same abnormalities in Cam's tests that he had discovered in Doug's, so he put the second child on magnesium oxide. Still, nothing could be definitely proven with only two children.

Months and days slipped by. Doug grew in spurts. The fine, birdlike appearance of his bones disappeared and became more rounded. He was still smaller than average, but he was growing stronger and sturdier. At the age of three, he stood for the first time on his tiny legs. And at three years, two months, and seventeen days, he walked alone. The Kellers cried with joy, then frantically hauled him off to their pediatrician and orthopedist, then to Denver to Dr. Solomons. Each place they echoed the same triumphant cry. "Look! Our child can walk!"

All that summer, Doug walked, and the sessions with Dr. Solomons continued. But unfortunately, in September, Doug suffered a broken leg—his first break since a fractured right arm at six weeks. Becky and Charles were crestfallen. They had been so sure he was getting better. Only seven weeks in a cast, then seven weeks out of it, and Doug was walking despite warnings that he might never walk again. Much of that winter was spent indoors, exercising and regaining lost strength. Entire mornings were spent on the floor kicking arms and legs amid protests and laughter. The housework and chores could wait. This was more important.

Cam wasn't as lucky. Most of his winter was being spent at Fitzsimmons Hospital. Infections and complications followed surgery. To cheer him and his mother, Becky often went to visit. While at the hospital one late February day, Beverly showed Becky my *Redbook* article.

"Her name is Gemma Geisman, and she lives in Ohio," Beverly told her. "I've already written to her. Maybe you'd like to write too."

After leaving the hospital, Becky headed for a newsstand to buy her own copy of the magazine. She read the article before going home, then reread it to Charles after arriving home.

"I was sick inside," she told me, "knowing that someone else had known the defeat and despair we had known. By evening, the sick feeling had turned into a desperate need to somehow reach you to tell you that there was hope for Mike. More than anything, I wanted to share that small glimmer of hope with you."

Chapter Twelve

From the seeds of sadness, a new family was conceived, and it grew quickly in love and understanding.

One afternoon, I was called to the telephone to take a long-distance call from Mississippi. Over the wire, I heard a breathless, excited voice. "Thank heavens, I found you! Until I read your article, I thought I was the only woman with a child like Joey. I've never known anyone else with this terrible disease. Please tell me more about Mike. Does he sit? Does he stand? Did he ever walk? Please tell me. My little Joey is only two, and I need to know what's ahead."

I hesitated. What could I really tell her? I knew so little about OI. Yet I felt compelled to tell her some of the positive things I had yearned to hear when Mike had been only two.

"Are you still there?" she asked, frantic that we may have been disconnected.

"I'm still here," I murmured as I groped to find the right words. "First, tell me who you are and where you live. There's so much to tell. Maybe it would be best if I wrote to you."

"Oh no!" she quickly replied. "I mean, yes, I'd like you to write, but there is so much I want to know *now*. Can we talk? That is, if you have a few minutes?"

"You can have all the time you want," I said and settled back in my chair to listen.

"My name is Joanne," she began. "I live in a small town near Tupelo, Mississippi, with my husband, Bo, and our three boys, Jamey, Joey, and Jon." Her voice trembled as she added, "Joey's so small, so fragile!"

"Mike is small and fragile too," I hastened to reassure her. "But we've found a place, Shriners Hospital in Chicago, where surgeons were able to straighten his legs and make them stronger. He even walked for a short time."

Gasping with pleasure, she cried, "Oh please, tell me more!"

I laughed. "Are you sure you want to hear all this?"

"Every bit of it," she replied.

"The first time Mike was admitted to Shriners, he was there for six months. It was tough having him so far away from home, but the long stay was necessary for him to have 'roddings' done on both of his femurs and tibias."

She admitted having heard the medical terms for bones that orthopedists use—terms that become so familiar to parents of children with OI. But she had never heard of rodding surgery. So I explained it to her the best I could.

I finished, saying, "The second time Mike was at Shriners for roddings, he stayed eight long months. But it was worth it. The day he was discharged, he walked down the long hospital corridor to meet us."

"That's incredible! We were told that Joey would never walk. Do you think he might someday?"

I couldn't lie to her. "Mike doesn't walk anymore," I confessed. "His legs simply couldn't support his body weight, even with the rods in them. So he's back in his wheelchair. However, he does everything but walk."

"Joey does too," she confided. "He sits up and hops on his little bottom, and I do mean little. He weighs only sixteen pounds. He goes all over the house by himself. He puts puzzles together, builds with blocks, and does everything a child his age can do. He's even beginning to pull himself up, but his strength is all in his arms. There's so little in his legs."

"You're lucky," I told her. "Joey's still young. With roddings and exercise, maybe he can learn to walk. Who knows, maybe a cure will be discovered in time for him."

Perhaps sensing that I was envious about time being on their side, she switched the topic to an observation she had made. "You know, it's uncanny how much Joey looks like Mike in the magazine snapshot. They could be brothers. Why is it that they look so much alike?"

I explained what Dr. Sofield had told us about how the unique characteristics of OI often resulted in remarkable resemblances among those affected. By now, it was clear to me that most of the families hadn't been aware of the look-alike factor until Mike's picture had appeared with my article.

We chatted for a while longer about other similarities; then finally, she said, "Gemma, just talking to you has helped so much. You will write, won't you?"

I assured her that I would write and send her information about Shriners and rodding surgery.

On the heels of Joanne's phone call came more letters and phone calls from other mothers of OI children who wanted to share their experiences and offer their support.

From Exeter, New Hampshire, Barbara St. Amour wrote, "I've just finished reading *My Prison of Dreams*, and I just had to tell you how much it meant to me. Although we are hundreds of miles apart, we have lived through many similar days. My name is Barbara, and our son, Gregg, who will be eleven in March, has the same condition as Mike. I have never written to anyone about my problem, but I know *you* will listen. Your experiences seem so much like mine. Please help me to understand this disease."

A dialogue developed quickly between Barbara and I. We were about the same age, had both been reared in small New England towns, and shared the same ethnic and religious backgrounds. More important, though, was the fact that our emotions had taken the same dreadful course. Sharing this information became incredibly therapeutic for both of us.

Down-to-earth, cheerful letters from Traverse City, Michigan, came to brighten my life. From practical Midge Peck, I learned to make new adjustments. "I have a son Mark who is like Mike," she wrote. "And I feel that your story is my story with few alterations. Mark weighs only twenty-eight pounds with full leg braces. He is in the sixth grade and has a teaching telephone hookup with the school. This allows him to participate fully in all classroom activities, and he loves it. I take him to school for assemblies and parties. He so enjoys being with his classmates.

"Mark has had rodding surgery and stands up inside a feeding table during school to reinforce his legs. He also has a tricycle he rides daily to develop his leg muscles."

The standing table, the teaching telephone, and the tricycle were new ideas that interested me very much. If at all possible, Mike would have them too. Without losing any time, I wrote to Midge for the details. She responded that the standing table had originally been a child's feeding table with a seat in the center. The seat was removed, and it had become a standing table that provided some protection from falling and had plenty of table space for books and papers. Enclosed was a brochure about the teaching telephone and a photo of Mark on his tricycle.

The teaching telephone appeared to be exactly what Mike needed. During my talks with school administrators, Mike's need for regular classroom participation had often been discussed, but never been solved. Since they wouldn't admit him to regular school, they agreed that a teaching telephone might be the next best thing. When the following school term began, Mike was no longer a class of one, thanks to Midge.

The standing table would have to wait until we could find a way to strengthen Mike's legs a bit more. Perhaps a small tricycle was the solution. Still, it frightened us to think what might happen to Mike while riding it. Was it too much to expect a child who couldn't walk to ride a tricycle? Maybe Mark's condition wasn't as severe as Mike's. It was a daring idea, but maybe it would work, make Mike's legs stronger.

On his twelfth birthday, we surrendered to the idea and bought Mike a small bright red tricycle. Like me, he was thrilled with the idea, but was worried about trying it. It took only a bit of coaxing, however, before he agreed to let Dick put him on the seat so he could get the feel of it. He looked so small, so scared, and I wanted to pull him off. Instead, trying to be calm, I placed my arms around him in a symbolic, protective circle and urged him to try pedaling. With much concentrated effort, and with the other children cheering him on, he strained to push the pedals down and make them go. It took time and a lot of huffing and puffing, but finally, he made it around the kitchen table unaided. When he stopped, we were all as exhausted as he was, but Mike was hooked. Soon, he was doing engine noises, like the race cars at Indianapolis, as he pedaled his hundred laps a day around the kitchen table.

To me, these new ideas were like miracles in themselves. My mounting jubilation about everything I was learning was something that I felt had to be shared. So I bought a stock of carbon paper and began sending letter copies to everyone on my growing mailing list.

At about this same time, I added Renee Gardner of Huntsville, Alabama, to the list. The bright promise of Renee's friendship shone through her first letter. She had a nine-year-old son, Donny, who had OI; and in her gentle, Southern manner, she offered me hope and encouragement.

Her story was not unlike the others, yet I found that she added more positiveness to the telling of it. From the beginning of our relationship, she stressed optimism and faith. She'd had bad experiences like the rest of us, but she chose not to dwell on them. Her letters were full of daily accomplishments and small battles won. These qualities endeared her to me, so I welcomed her invitation to correspond.

Much to our mutual delight, Renee and I discovered that we had other things in common besides OI. We were both aspiring authors who loved to read. From the beginning, our letters were filled with little notes like "Have you read *Earth Shine* by Ann Morrow Lindbergh? I loved it!" Or "I'm still dreaming of becoming a writer, you've made a beginning as one."

I found her letters heartwarming; she found mine inspiring. Thus, we soon became a mutual admiration society of two. It was fun and exhilarating to know someone so much the same, yet so different. Our friendship added much to our lives.

In my letters to my newfound friends, I told them about Becky Keller and Dr. Solomons and about their ongoing search for more children with OI to join in the research project. All wanted to know more.

To Becky, I wrote, "I've asked all the mothers on my mailing list to contact Dr. Solomons if they're interested in participating in his research. Also, what do you think about forming some sort of mothers' club so we can continue to share ideas and help each other?"

"Your idea of a mothers' club sounds great," she answered. "How do you propose to do it?"

I replied. "I don't know. Let's think about it."

In another letter, Becky volunteered, "I majored in journalism and know something about putting out a paper. Maybe a little newspaper or newsletter is the answer. We could pool our knowledge of OI and share it with the others. If you're willing, I am!"

"I'm more than willing," I wrote back. "Let's do it!"

My desire to provide information about OI to other parents and Becky's efforts to encourage the study of the disease were enough reasons for us to want to find a way of communicating what information we had to others.

With that goal in mind, our lives became filled with a compulsion to learn everything we could about OI. From Renee, Midge, and the other mothers, we began to garner information about medical treatments our children had or had not received.

Barbara St. Amour, for instance, had been concerned about their family doctor's reliance on sedatives to soothe Gregg's pain. Each time he saw Gregg, the doctor had strengthened the sedation, until at ten months, he was taking doses of Demerol twice a day. At nineteen months, his pain had grown excessively worse, and the effectiveness of the medicine had lessened. Barbara told us, "By then, I found myself desperately pleading with God to hurry up and take Gregg. Maybe we were naive, but it didn't occur to us to question our doctor or seek other medical opinions. We had been told point-blank that it was senseless to hope that Gregg would live. We'd also been told with finality that there was no medical help available. Still, we had to find a way to lessen our baby's pain while he was with us."

Word of their plight spread around town; then one evening, a tall dark man, dressed in a business suit, had come knocking at their door. He introduced himself as a chiropractor and said that friends of theirs had sent him. "I'd like to help your baby if I can," he told them.

Barbara and George were skeptical that a small broken body could be helped by chiropractic manipulations, but they listened to what he had to say, and before he left that evening, they had agreed to let him come twice a week on a trial basis even though they knew that their doctor wouldn't approve. "Gregg never had another sedative after that night. Doc, as we fondly called him, came twice a week for three years without pay. He was gentle and didn't use the conventional adjustments a chiropractor uses in his daily work but, instead, used conservative adjustments with no forceful pressure. After three years, the visits were down to once a month, then only as needed. I know this is against the views of medical doctors, and I don't advocate it for other babies with OI," Barbara wrote, "but for us, it was the only help."

Years later, the St. Amours again were brutally reminded that there was no medical help for Gregg. They had left him with a family member to go camping with their other children when they got a phone call that Gregg had apparently broken his leg. Thinking that one of the other children in the family had been injured, the doctor they contacted to meet them at the emergency room said, "I'll send an ambulance over right away, and we'll have him admitted."

Finding this unusual, Barbara said, "Doctor, it's Gregg."

After a long, awkward pause, the doctor had responded, "Barbara, you know there's nothing we can do for Gregg. I'll come over and give him something for the pain if you want me to."

Mike's condition, when he had been released from the Indiana hospital several weeks after his birth, and Barbara's stories infuriated and frustrated us all. These horrendous experiences would never happen to anyone else's child, we vowed. Not if we could help it.

From Midge, we learned that after having four girls and before Mark, she had given birth to another little boy named Bruce. The doctors told them that Brucie had been born with no skull and that his entire head was soft, like the soft spot on a normal baby's head. He said that all they could do was take him home and care for him the best they could.

"I guess I knew from the very beginning that Brucie would be with us for just a little while," Midge recalled. "He was so small, so fragile. But it didn't matter to me. I held him in my arms and nursed him and loved him. When he was nearly five months old, he even laughed out loud, and I was overjoyed at his alert and bright responses. But one night, I awakened to the sound of his labored breathing and knew before I called the doctor that something was terribly wrong."

The doctor ordered the baby to the hospital, and when they arrived, he was immediately given oxygen. "I felt as I handed him over to the nurse that I wouldn't be holding him in my arms again. But I didn't give up. For a couple of days, I watched him cling to life while we clung to hope. On the second day, he rallied a little and seemed to have moments when he knew me. That evening, when the doctor reported that the congestion was gone and that the baby had smiled for him, we were all so excited."

However, the next day, as Midge was readying herself to go to the hospital, the phone rang. It was the doctor calling to say that Brucie had died. "It's for the best," the doctor had said in an attempt to comfort her.

When Midge discovered she was pregnant again, she was terrified. Her doctor tried to reassure her, but he too was worried. So it was with relief that he felt the new baby's head during delivery. It appeared hard and normal, with a well-formed skull. Moments later, however, he knew that his relief had been premature. The Peck's newborn was a mass of broken bones.

This time, there were no explanations from medical textbooks needed. In a barely audible voice, the doctor told them, "You have another son. I'm sorry, but he has OI too."

"How can this be?" I wrote after hearing Midge's story. "*We* weren't told that OI is inherited. In fact, we were told it was a fluke of nature that wouldn't be repeated and to go ahead and have more children. Becky was told *not* to have other children because OI was genetic in origin. Now this from Midge! We need to find out what is fact and what isn't!"

Renee's experiences with the medical community had been more positive. She and Don had been told from the start that OI was a genetic defect, yet they had decided to take a chance and have another child—a healthy son they had named Scott.

"We had understanding pediatricians and interested orthopedic men who urged us to try ordinary things in unordinary ways to help our baby," Renee wrote.

With the help of therapists, who encouraged them to hold and touch their child, the Gardners tried to develop each and every capability to the fullest. Feeling no shame for some impairment that was no fault of theirs, they harbored no guilt feelings about Donny and so displayed him to the world with pride.

"Friends and family were amazed, sometimes even puzzled, by our broad-minded attitudes, yet the interest of onlookers was genuine. Maybe it was this openness that encouraged our doctors to seek out ways and means of helping. Some went out of their way to devote extra time and study, learning all they could about OI so they could help Donny."

The positive medical attention Mike had received at Shriners, Dr. Solomons's interest in Doug Keller's well-being, and Donny Gardner's success in spurring doctors to learn more about OI was the kind of information we wanted to share with others in the medical community. To parents, we wanted to say, "It's okay to hold and cuddle your breakable baby. Midge and Renee did it!" Or "Try getting your baby in the water. Splashing is great therapy."

Having all this new and exciting information about daily living with OI made us realize that we were accumulating more knowledge about the disorder than the so-called experts had ever been able to give us. Excited by this discovery, we could hardly wait to get the presses rolling with the very first to be published, exclusively OI newsletter.

Chapter Thirteen

Dr. Solomons didn't waste any time answering the mothers who wrote to him. "Yes, I would like to include Mike in my studies and prepare him for testing and treatment," he told me. Cautioning that his findings were not to be considered a cure, he said he had isolated several factors of the disorder and begun experimental treatment with magnesium oxide. His letter went on to say that he was born in South Africa and had done his postgraduate work training in the United States and Canada, where he had investigated OI and other childhood diseases.

Reading this, I was beside myself with joy. For the first time since Mike's birth, there was hope that someday a cure would be found. I phoned our family doctor and made preparations to begin the many blood and urine tests Dr. Solomons needed. It all seemed too good to be true. And it was.

Only a few days after receiving Dr. Solomons's letter, the entire project came to a halt, at least where Mike was concerned. A letter from the staff at Shriners informed us that Mike had been scheduled for more rodding surgery that very week. The frustration I felt is beyond description. Once again, our plans to help Mike were being thwarted.

"What about Dr. Solomons's research? What about the new treatment? It's not fair to be stopped before we can even get started," I lamented. With Dick's encouragement, and determined to save the situation somehow, I wrote to Dr. Solomons, asking him to postpone Mike's tests until after his surgery. I received a very quick reply.

"Please ask Mike's surgeons to cooperate with me," he wrote. "I would very much like to have chips of Mike's bone. These and blood samples before and after surgery would help my research greatly."

His response reignited my jubilation. Shriners had been the center for rodding surgery for years. Wouldn't the staff there be aware of hundreds of children who might benefit from Dr. Solomons's research? Here was a chance to find lots of participants for his vital research. Armed with all the information and very determined to get Mike involved as soon as possible, I would insist that they send some of his blood and bone chips to Dr. Solomons.

Soon after Mike had been admitted, I asked to speak with Dr. Millar. This was a bold demand for me to make, for even though he had performed most of Mike's surgery, I really didn't know him well. I didn't have long to worry; I was politely informed that he wasn't there.

This was not unusual. Dr. Millar was a busy surgeon who spent many hours in the operating room. Admissions were routinely processed by the residents and nurses. Reluctantly, I told my exciting news to a somewhat skeptical resident. After hearing me out, he finally agreed to give my letters from Dr. Solomons to Dr. Millar, cautioning me all the while not to put too much stock in research that might prove fruitless.

I left Mike that day with a very heavy heart, thinking that this was probably the end of another wild and marvelous dream, that nobody would listen. But I was wrong. Instead, it turned out to be the beginning of something quite wonderful.

Mike had surgery in May, and during the remainder of his hospital stay, we visited him nearly every weekend. On each of these occasions, I prodded whichever resident was making the Sunday afternoon rounds. "Do you know if Dr. Millar wrote to Dr. Solomons? Were the bone chips sent as we asked? And what about the blood and urine samples? Were they sent? Do you know anything . . . anything at all?" Every question I asked was answered with a blank look or an I-don't-know response. No one could or would tell me anything.

Still without a word being said about the research, Mike was discharged in early July, looking like a pale little turtle in a plaster shell. Only his head and shoulders, arms and toes protruded from his large body cast. Due to the semireclining position of the cast, he had to sit that way and couldn't participate in the usual whiffle ball games that summer. So to while away the hot, humid days, he and I took to spending a lot of time, sitting in the shade together, talking.

Mike never missed much of what went on around him, and he told me that he was positive the doctors had taken blood and urine samples and sent the requested bone chips to Dr. Solomons. "Most of the time, the doctors discuss us as if we're not even there," he said. "But I listen to everything they say. It's my body they're messing with, and I want to know every single thing they take out and put back into it. I'm *positive* they sent everything Dr. Solomons wanted."

Encouraged by what Mike told me, I waited out his cast removal appointment writing letters in an effort to find out more about the research going on at the University of Colorado.

In August, Renee wrote, "I took Donny in for a checkup today. Since he is now on magnesium oxide, Dr. Foley likes to keep a close watch on him. She says that he seems to be in better health than when he started. I certainly have seen a physical change in Donny. It's possible that it's due to the clearing up of the constipation problem, but whatever it is, we are really happy with his progress at the present time. The last few years, we had been getting scared that nothing more could be done for him. Now this!"

Working with Dr. Solomons, Dr. Foley had put Donny on magnesium oxide on an individual patient basis. I was thrilled that he was doing so well because of it.

Mark Peck wasn't on MgO yet, but he kept Mike amused about their attempts to get it through their doctor. In his comical letters, he brought a spark of brightness to Mike's difficult months of convalescing.

Becky, who had an inside line on the research at Colorado general, wrote that she had heard that some patients from Shriners had recently been or soon would be prescribed magnesium oxide. Puzzled and irritated at not having been informed of this, I wrote to Dr. Solomons.

He replied that there was a possibility that some patients at Shriners would participate in his research and be prescribed MgO. His letter had an air of subdued eagerness and guarded caution, and he advised us to question Dr. Millar concerning Mike's participation in the project.

I was happy to hear that Dr. Solomons and Dr. Millar were in touch. Yet I worried that my son was being left out. The day Mike's cast was finally removed, I pleaded with the resident sawing the cast. "*Please* tell me if Dr. Millar sent Mike's blood samples and bone chips to Dr. Solomons. I can't bear not knowing anymore!"

The youthful doctor appeared surprised that I knew anything at all about the Colorado study. He was thoughtful for a moment then, at last, he said, "Yes, he did. We're going to draw more blood today and send it for further tests. Ask Dr. Millar when you come back for the regular clinic. He'll tell you all about it."

Mike smirked. "I told you, Mom. The people around here are vampires. They can't resist any chance to draw blood!"

The young resident snickered at Mike's remark as he left to find his next victim. Thankful for what little information he had given us, we drove home in a more positive frame of mind. Waiting for the regular clinic day wouldn't be half as hard now that we knew something was being done.

In October, I was delighted to see that Dr. Millar was making the rounds of the cubicles and seeing the children himself. When finally he entered the compartment where we waited, he smiled at me in the quizzical manner I came to know so well and nodded hello.

Peering at me through his wire-rimmed glasses, he said, "So I hear you have a lot of questions for me?" then turned away to examine Mike's arms and legs.

Smiling nervously at his back, I replied, "You bet I do."

He turned on his stool, settled himself against the examining table, lifted his eyebrows in my direction, and waited. Boldly, I said, "I want to know the results of your contacts with Dr. Solomons."

Smiling to himself, he tapped his knee with the packet of medical records he was holding and pondered what to say. Absently, he toyed with the buttons on his blue medical coat and gave me another appraising glance. "You're the one who informed us of Dr. Solomons's work, aren't you?"

"Yes, I brought you his letters when Mike was in for surgery, and I've been trying to find out ever since what, if anything, has been done about getting involved in his research."

Smiling broadly, he said, "Well, then, I guess you have a right to know. I did what you wanted. I got in touch with Dr. Solomons. I even flew to Denver to see him. I flew out there, had dinner with him, and went over his research. I was very impressed. I think maybe he can help these children. I've asked the Chicago Shriners Unit to participate in and help finance a two-year research program with Dr. Solomons. If it's approved, we'll be setting up a clinic soon."

"And Mike will be included?" I asked, barely above a whisper.

"You'll hear from us as soon as the details can be worked out. And of course, Mike will be included! He and several other children have already had some tests, so if we go ahead with the research, he'll be one of the first to go on magnesium oxide."

That was the end of the questions and answers for that day. Turning his attention back to Mike, Dr. Millar examined his legs again, then beamed at the x-rays of his pride and joy—the new telescoping rod he had recently implanted in them.

As he left the room, I said, "Thanks for everything you're doing."

With a light wave of his hand, he dismissed my thanks and said, "I'm doing it for the kids. Let's hope it does them some good."

In mid-January, a letter with this message came from Dr. Millar:

Dear parents:

As some of you know, we have been working with Dr. Clive Solomons of the University of Colorado on the problems of brittle bones. Dr. Solomons's experience suggests that by giving children with osteogenesis imperfecta magnesium oxide, that the bones can be hardened up to some degree. There has been no evidence of dangerous side effects of this treatment in the small number of patients who have received it. It is our hope to place approximately thirty of our patients on this type of therapy. This study will cover a period of at least two years.

In order that this program will be clearly understood by everybody involved, we plan to hold a special clinic on the twenty-third of January between 9 and 10 a.m. At that time, additional laboratory tests will be obtained both from the parents and children. In addition, details will be gone over with you personally concerning future laboratory tests and medication

Would you please indicate on the enclosed card if you will be able to attend this clinic.

Below his signature, Dr. Millar had scrawled, "Mrs. Geisman, the seed for this was planted by you. Thanks. E. Millar."

I read and reread the letter countless times; and as I did so, I marveled that this time, the seed had sprouted out of hopefulness rather than out of sadness. And I sat down to write the good news to all my friends.

Chapter Fourteen

January 23, 1969—a day to remember. Dick, Mike, and I woke up in the wee hours of the morning to the insistent buzzing of the alarm clock. Quietly, we crawled out of bed, got dressed, and tiptoed down the stairs so as not to wake the other members of the family who still slept soundly. Grandma had come to spend the night so she could be with the children. We walked past her sleeping on the sofa, and she stirred but didn't wake up.

I hadn't wanted to go to sleep at all. Anticipation fluttered like butterflies in my stomach, for I knew that I would soon witness the rebirth of hope in a group of parents and children. For myself, I wanted more than ever to have this second chance to do something wonderful for Mike, and I feared that if I slept, I would wake up and find that it was only a dream.

During the ride to Chicago, my happiness showed me the world in a new light. Everything seemed astonishingly more beautiful, more brilliant. The lone morning star seemed lower than usual—almost within reach. Light floated softly out of the darkness, revealing a bright new world filling quickly with awakening life. In my mind, I heard a whisper of words I'd read somewhere and stored away. "Today is the first day of the rest of your life," the words proclaimed. And indeed, at that moment, it did seem as if a new life was about to begin for Mike, and for many other children we didn't even know.

We arrived at Shriners a half hour early to discover that only one other family had beat us there. A young girl and her parents were reading a sign on the clinic door—a sign directing us to another door. As we walked around the building with them, they seemed guarded and spoke only when spoken to. Other than snapshots, I hadn't seen many children with OI, so I examined the beautiful, pale blonde child with the large blue eyes. She appeared to be near average in size, had few deformities, and walked well with crutches. I remember thinking, *They're lucky! She looks so normal!* And I couldn't help but wonder why her young parents had such strained and worried expressions on their faces.

Thirteen-year-old Mike was making his own observations. "Cute, isn't she? I wonder how old she is?" he whispered to his dad and me.

In the empty waiting room, we sat on folding chairs, facing the other family. At first, we exchanged the usual small talk that strangers make about the weather and traffic conditions; then we grew silent as other families began to arrive. It was almost as if we were at a look-alike convention. It was uncanny the way so many of the children resembled one another. Among the thirty or so attending, we saw every conceivable form of the disorder.

Some of the youngsters were so average in size and looks, it was hard to believe that they were affected at all. Then there were others who looked like little men wearing the bodies of infants. Many had heads that were flatter and more deformed than Mike's had ever been. Some couldn't sit or lift up their heads and had to be brought to the clinic in reclining seats or portable cribs. With a measure of consolation, I estimated Mike to be an in-between case. Not as severely affected as some, but not as normal looking as others.

At first, every parent and child group remained aloof, isolated within themselves, as if alone on an island. This kind of detachment was a protection device that we'd all learned to use to shield our children from public reaction. It hadn't yet dawned on any of the others that it wasn't needed here in this particular setting where everyone was affected by osteogenesis imperfecta.

I looked openly into some of the faces, but out of habit, their eyes quickly averted mine. I wanted to say, "Don't look away from me. I've been there too. I have the same problems, the same fears." But all I did was smile lamely. I couldn't bring myself to say the desired words. Sharing personal histories face-to-face, I discovered, didn't come as easily as it had in letters or over the phone.

Mike, on the other hand, was doing a lot of news sharing of his own. I noticed him whispering with some of the kids I assumed he knew from past hospitalizations. Once he was finished saying whatever it was he was telling, I noticed some of the other children going back to their parents to whisper in *their* ears. The result inevitably made them glance in our direction.

When, finally, I was able to corner Mike to ask what he was up to, he grinned. "I told them that if it hadn't been for my mom and me, this big research thing would never have happened."

Unlike the parents, the children curiously examined one another, and before long, they were talking and laughing together as if they had been friends forever. Their camaraderie eventually began to evoke a slow response from some of the adults in the room. Tentatively, they smiled at one another, then at us. How they must have wondered about all the specifics of what was about to happen, and how could they so cleverly suppress their eagerness to ask. I knew all about it, and I was practically jumping out of my skin!

All the children were weighed, measured, and photographed for the record. When Mike's picture was taken wearing only his undershorts, he quipped, "Is this for *Playboy*?" The laughter that followed was a great tension reliever.

When the parents had filled out individual questionnaires and undergone blood tests with their children, we were reassembled in the clinic room to listen to Dr. Millar and his assistants explain the research program. Medical personnel were bustling about, taking pictures of the history-making event, and setting up charts and blackboards with detailed information.

At last, Dr. Millar sauntered in, wearing his long blue medical coat. He cleared his throat, and instantly, the room grew silent.

He began by saying that sometime ago, a mother had written in a national magazine about her experiences raising an OI child. (Proud beams from Mike and Dick flashed in my direction.) As a result of the article, Dr. Millar continued, he had become aware of some research being done by Dr. Clive Solomons at the University of Colorado Medical Center.

Dr. Solomons had isolated a substance, pyrophosphate, which was present in high concentration in the blood of patients with OI. "The substance could be used as an indicator of the genetic defect that underlies the formation of brittle bones," he explained. Dr. Solomons had found that when magnesium oxide was administered, it lowered the pyrophosphate and allowed for a more normal action of calcium and phosphorous metabolism.

After the explanations were over, a few parents ventured vague questions. The gist of their questions led me to believe that the reality of what was happening hadn't yet set in. It would take more time for them to absorb it all.

In February, the children returned to the clinic for additional testing. At that time, we were given a supply of magnesium oxide capsules that would last until the April clinic. (Mike was to begin with six capsules a day.) In addition, parents were to keep temperature charts and menu sheets to establish the food habits and normal temperature of each child.

At the April clinic, nearly all the children showed increases in their weight and height. Mike had gained four pounds and grown a whole inch! Never had he grown so fast. His sweating and constipation—also symptoms—had diminished. All the parents were thrilled.

The July clinic was more routine. By then, we were getting used to blood tests and chart keeping. Once again, most of the children showed definite improvement, but this time, it was less dramatic. There is a spurt of growth, we were told, shortly after magnesium oxide is first administered, then a small lag, then slower but steady progress. A side benefit of the clinic was that now, the parents were beginning to open up to one another about their children and the problems they had encountered caring for them. This was a delightful turn of events. It was like witnessing a flower bloom in slow motion.

In between clinics, I kept our mothers' group posted with long, descriptive letters, telling them about the progress of the research and about the children and parents I had met. They benefited from and enjoyed the letters very much.

From New Hampshire, Barbara wrote, "Even though we can't attend the clinics, it certainly is great to be able to correspond with someone who does. Your letters are always so welcomed. They have helped me understand that others have the same problems we have."

"I'm glad there is improvement for Mike and the other kids," Midge said. "I have so much hope for Mark now that I've heard about the clinics. We're waiting for our doctor to make arrangements to send Mark's blood samples to Dr. Solomons. I can hardly wait!"

From Renee, I heard, "As I finished the supper dishes tonight, I looked out my kitchen window to see Donny sitting in the swing with such a happy expression on his face as he pumped himself. This is a small example of the many things that have happened to him this summer. I have truly wondered if his newfound confidence comes from our hopes or from sharing with other families' problems similar to ours. Perhaps it is both. Sometimes God answers our prayers in ways we never expect. The beginning was a story in a magazine."

I was touched by Renee's words, and for a fleeting moment, I thought, *I should write to the editors of Redbook to tell them what's happened.*

"Oh, how well I remember those test charts and menu watching!" Becky responded when she heard what we were doing. "For months, I had to weigh Doug's food to the ounce. And those blood tests! How we dreaded them!"

These words reminded me that Becky and her small son were the real pioneers in this research. Unknowingly, they had paved the way for the Chicago clinics. In characteristic form, Becky hitched this afterthought to the end of her letter: "Gemma, how about a follow-up article for *Redbook*?"

I laughed when I read it. It was amazing how often we operated on the same wavelength.

One early June morning, I sat at my typewriter and began to outline an article for the magazine. I worked all morning on an opening, but nothing I wrote sounded right. The next morning, I ripped up my first attempts and started over again. But not far into the piece, a letter came to destroy the rosy glow of success I was trying to convey. It was from an eighteen-year-old girl who had just heard about my original article.

"I can't tell you how hopeful my husband and I became after we read your article and realized that there were others trying to cope with the same problems. Our little Jeffery is only a year old, and we've nearly lost him several times."

The letter continued with all the usual questions about OI—but at the end, there was a postscript: "I'm sorry for the delay in getting this letter to you, but Jeffery died at one o'clock today, June 5. I hope this doesn't keep you from writing to me, telling me everything you know. I would still like my questions answered."

Through tear-filled eyes, I gazed at the delicate writing on the pale yellow paper and marveled at the inner strength of this young woman to have been able to finish this letter at all on the day her baby had died. My happiness at what I had been doing for children with OI dissolved quickly as I realized that the good news was too late for little Jeffery.

Throwing away my scanty article openers, I began a letter of condolence to the youthful parents.

Six weeks later, around mid-July, I decided to give the article another try. It was hot and humid in my small writing room, and the ambition to write a long, detailed article was practically nonexistent. Close by, a large pile of letters waited to be answered. Letters were so much easier for me. Why couldn't I just write *Redbook* a letter, combining what had resulted from the first article with a note of thanks for making it happen?

Rolling a clean sheet of paper into my typewriter, I began, "Dear editors of *Redbook*. Many dreams, like some stories, have an epilogue. Sometimes the dream continues, takes different shape, acquires new faces, and, at last, is no longer a dream but a real event bringing hope to many. That is what happened to me and my dream because of your magazine, and I would like to tell you about it."

Oblivious of the heat, I wrote for nearly two hours about everything that had happened. Several days later, I rewrote it and mailed it, satisfied to have finally thanked the editors properly.

Months passed, and before we knew it, it was clinic time again. I was very eager to attend the October clinic because I had advance information from Becky that Dr. Solomons would be there. He was to arrive a week ahead of the clinic date to make a detailed study of all the charts.

On the scheduled day, after the usual routine, Dr. Millar introduced him to the assembly. Dr. Solomons was an attractive man, probably in his early forties, with a soft-spoken South African English accent. He told us what a privilege it was for him to be able to work with us. Previously, he had known only a few children with OI, but since he had begun work with our large group, he had made strides in all aspects of his research. Already, some of his findings were being used to treat other childhood diseases.

Dr. Solomons said that the blood tests of our group had established his earlier findings and that all but three of the thirty-six children had shown improvement, and that these three were progressing at a slower rate.

He emphasized that his studies had not achieved a "cure" and that we should temper our great hopes to the reality of the situation.

When he had finished speaking, Dr. Solomons and Dr. Millar examined each child individually. When Mike's turn came, Dr. Millar introduced Dr. Solomons to me, saying, "This is the culprit who started all this!"

Dr. Solomons laughed. "I'm glad these mothers write and nag us. It encourages us to go on."

Everything Becky had told me about Dr. Solomons was true. He was obviously not only interested in the research, but in what we, the parents, had to say. What a good feeling it was to hear him and Dr. Millar talk about the research possibilities as they examined Mike. Even though we knew that scientific research offers no guarantees, it was enough for us just then to know that our children's bleak futures now mattered to someone willing to help us search for solutions.

It was the best of times, it was the worst of times, it was the age of wisdom, it was the age of foolishness, it was the epoch of belief, it was the epoch of incredulity, it was the season of Light, it was the season of Darkness, it was the spring of hope, it was the winter of despair. (*A Tale of Two Cities*, 1859)

THE EARLY YEARS

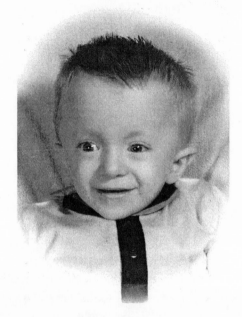

Mike at age one

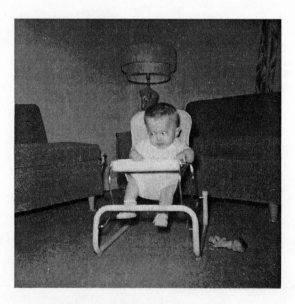

Mike sitting for the first time

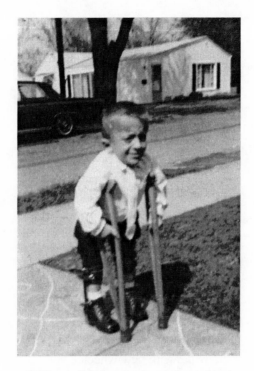

Mike walking only for a short time

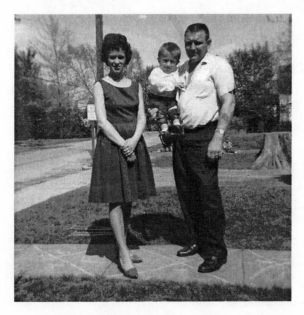

Gemma, Mike, Dick

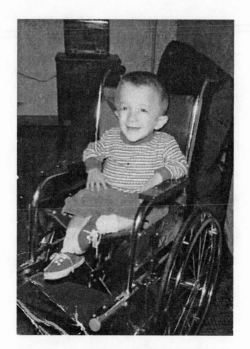

Mike with new wheelchair

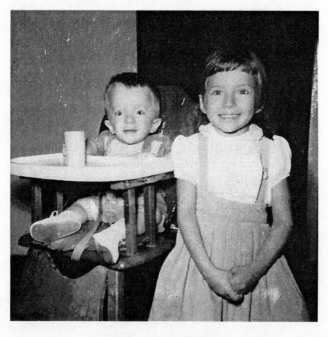

Mike and Cathy

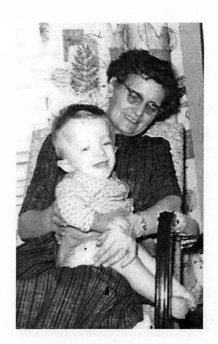

Mike and Grandma

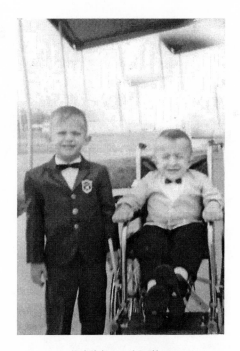

Dickie and Mike

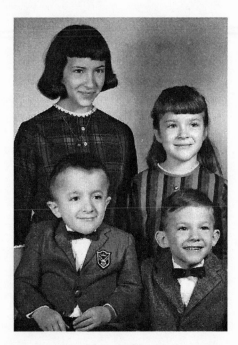

Mike and Dickie seated, Cathy and Cindy standing

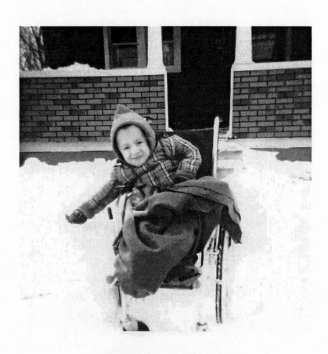

Mike playing in the snow

CHICAGO MEETING-APRIL 1970

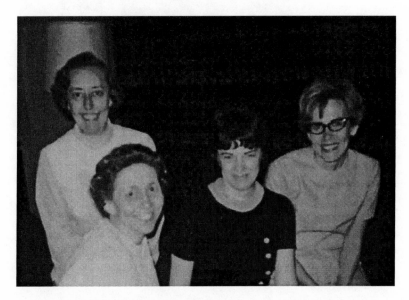

Becky Keller behind Midge Peck, Gemma Geisman, Renee
Gardner

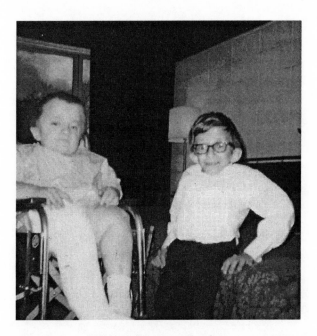

Mike and Donny Gardner

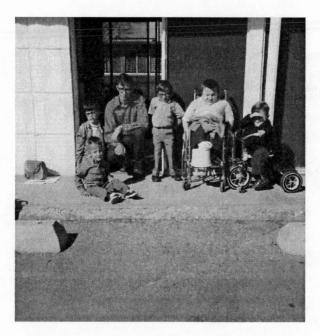

Doug Keller on the ground, Scott Gardner, Joe
Keller, Donny Gardner, Mike, and Mark Peck

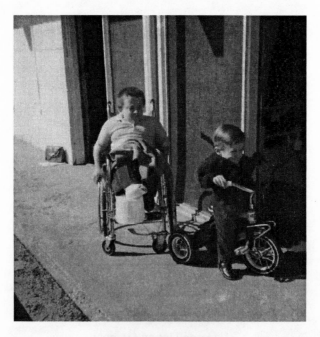

Mike and Mark Peck

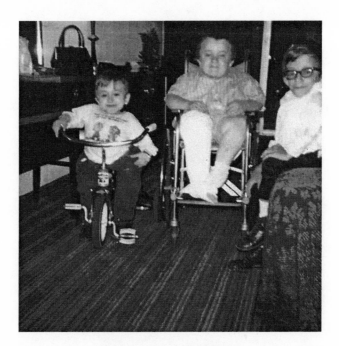

Mark, Mike and Donny

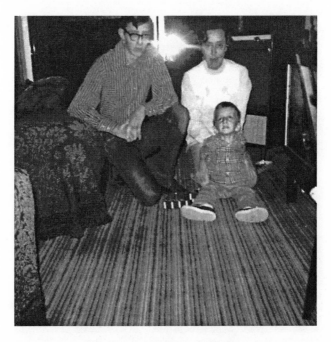

Joe, Becky and Doug Keller

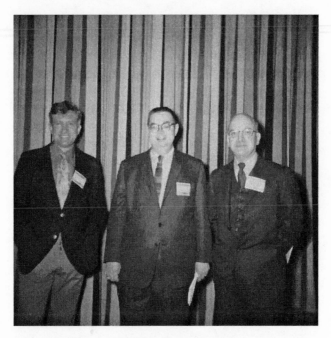

Dr. Clive Solomons, Dr. John Ott, Dr. Edward Millar

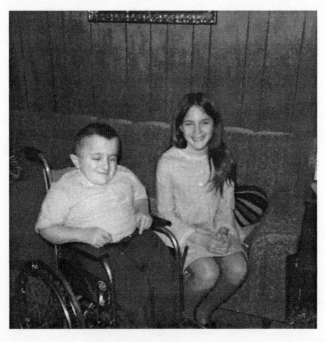

Mike and Cindy as teenagers

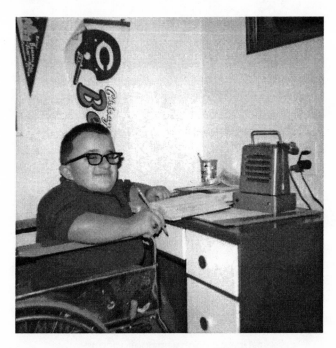

Mike going to high school on his intercom

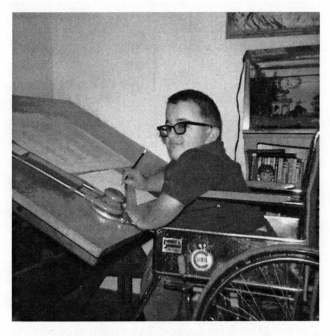

Mike at his drafting board

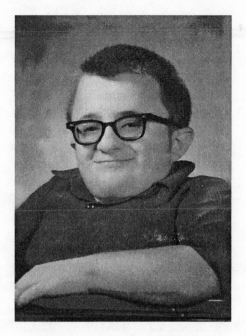

Mike's senior yearbook picture

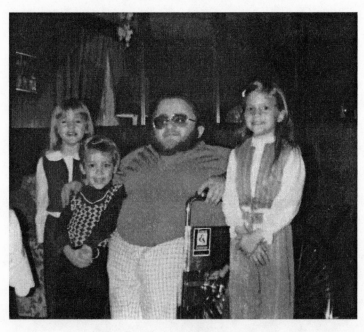

Mike at age 23 with his nephew, Ryan and nieces Emily and
Jennifer

SOME OF THE OI FAMILIES

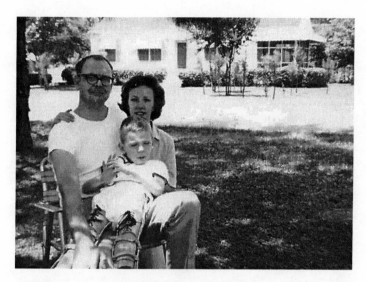

The Burdette family

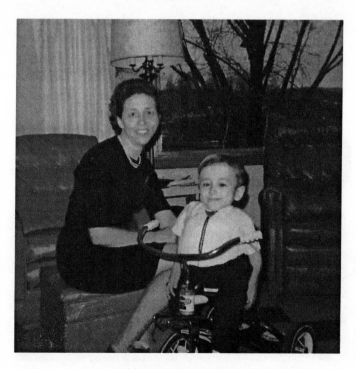

Midge and Mark Peck

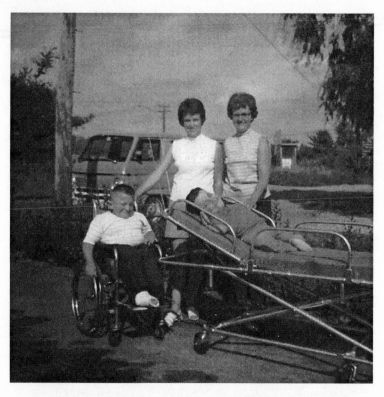

Mike and Gemma with Barbara and Gregg St. Amour

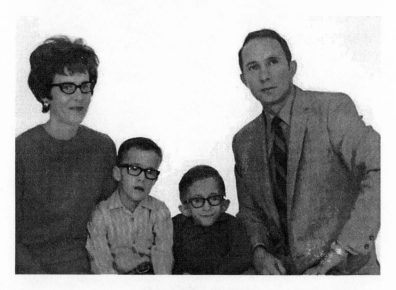

The Gardner family

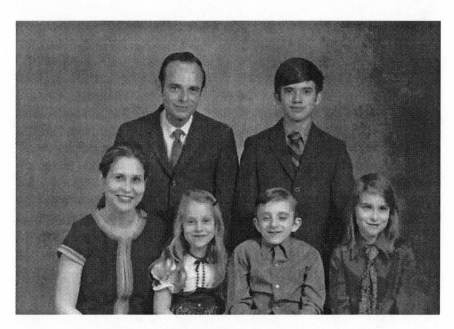

The McNeely family

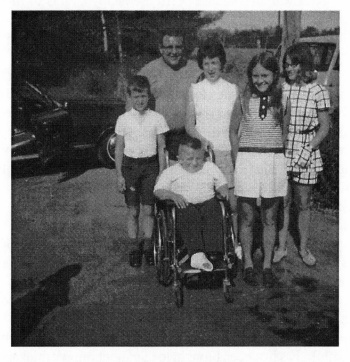

The Geisman family

Chapter Fifteen

Through my kitchen window, I saw a fat squirrel furtively burying treasure under a walnut tree and heard the happy shouts of my sons as they scrimmaged with neighborhood friends among the fallen leaves. Inside, Dick chatted with me while I cooked dinner, and the girls pored studiously over their new schoolbooks.

Only two weeks had passed since the October clinic, yet on that late afternoon in early November, I felt truly fulfilled. At last, our efforts and dreams were reaping a harvest. Numerous new friends enriched our lives. Mike was receiving promising medical attention, and our three other children were healthy and happy. I wanted or needed nothing more.

Suddenly, the phone rang noisily, sounding like a loud giggle in the quiet lull. I reached for it on the kitchen wall while I continued to stir the pudding on the stove with my free hand.

"Mrs. Geisman?" a friendly woman's voice asked, and before I could respond, she went on. "Mrs. Geisman, this is Dorothy Gallagher at *Redbook* magazine. I've just read your letter, and I think it's simply marvelous!"

I reached over to turn off the heat under the pudding and asked, "What letter?"

"Please forgive us, Mrs. Geisman," she continued. "But your letter, written last July, has just been brought to our attention. We think the events you described in it are wonderful, and we'd like to be able to publish it."

"Oh, *that* letter," I said, trying desperately to remember what I had written on that sultry summer day. "You want to publish it?"

"Yes, with your permission, we'd like to include it in the March issue as a special epilogue to your first story." She paused, then prodded, "Mrs. Geisman?"

"I'm not sure I remember what I wrote in that letter. It was months ago."

Because I had addressed the letter to the editors of *Redbook*, she explained, it had traveled around with piles of unsolicited articles until it had finally been discovered by a manuscript reader. After chatting a bit more, Ms. Gallagher and I agreed that I needed a few days to review my copy of the letter, after which time, we would talk again to iron out the details.

As I hung up, Dick very cautiously asked, "What was *that* all about?"

Still somewhat dumfounded, I answered, "*Redbook* wants to publish my letter."

"What letter?" he asked, giving me one of his "here we go again" looks.

I realized then that I hadn't mentioned sending what I had regarded as a routine thank-you letter. Becky was the only one I had told. Rather than try to explain it to him, I went to my filing cabinet and fished out the copy of the letter I had written that hot July day and gave it to him to read. When he was finished, he said, "No wonder *Redbook* wants to publish it. It's a great letter."

Days full of excitement and activity followed. I was in constant contact with *Redbook* editors, who plied me with questions and asked that I write an additional piece, detailing the October clinic and our meeting with Dr. Solomons to be incorporated with the original letter. Derived from the opening sentence of my letter, the finished piece would be fittingly titled "Epilogue to a Dream."

Editor in chief Sey Chassler wrote a nice note. "We are delighted to hear that *Redbook* was of some use, and we fully intend to use your new story in some specific way. Now that you know us by name, please write to us directly! With all best wishes. It is a personal joy to hear from you in this way."

William Hart, a senior editor, flew to Ohio to interview me. I need not have been nervous about meeting a big-time magazine editor for the first time. He immediately put me at ease. During the drive from his hotel to our house for lunch, he told us he was very anxious to meet Mike but otherwise said very little about my letter. After lunch, he spoke with Mike and visited his room where he was shown how the phone hookup with school worked. Later, alone in the quiet of my writing room, he asked me a few simple but direct questions. Then smiling, he said, "I have what I came for."

Outdoors, rain was falling in a gloomy downpour. But inside, the conversation was pleasant and relaxed. I asked a lot of questions about the workings of a magazine, and Mr. Hart encouraged me to keep writing. "You write well," he said. "You should write more." When I confessed that I had written a lot of things I had never dared to submit, he said, "To be successful, you must be persistent. Take those dusty manuscripts out of your files and desk drawers. Keep sending them out and never give up."

After he had gone, letters heralding the good news went out to my friends. All were delighted to learn that "our story," as they so aptly put it, would once again be appearing in this widely respected women's magazine.

At my request, and to ensure accuracy, Dr. Solomons and Dr. Millar were sent copies of the article before publication. I didn't want my letter to imply that a cure for osteogenesis imperfecta had been found, only that the search had begun.

In early January, I heard from Becky. "The newsletter is still on my mind," she said. "In fact, it is so much so that I finally invested in a newer typewriter—this one is only about forty years old! However, it does have sharper keys on it for cutting stencils, and I'm hoping that we can get this thing off the ground this spring. Send me all the addresses you have!"

"Why wait until spring?" I replied. "Let's do it now before my article comes out. That way, we'll be ready if there's any kind of response."

Without waiting to hear from Becky, I wrote the first issue as a one-page newsletter and gave it the grand title of "Mothers Association for OI."

"This is the first issue of the quarterly newsletter to be published by a group of mothers with one common goal—to help parents who have children with osteogenesis imperfecta," the newsletter began. The following was an item about Dr. Solomons's research, then another about the Shriners clinic. There was a plug for Dr. Solomons's published paper on OI and a mention of my forthcoming epilogue in *Redbook*. At the end of the page was a request for the names and addresses of all who wished to be on the mailing list. Bursting with pride, I mailed the first copy to Becky.

Within a few days, I received a stack of neatly mimeographed copies back from her with an attached letter. "Here they are! Aren't they beautiful?" I could almost see her beaming across the miles as I read, "I'm getting ready for an onslaught of mail," she wrote. "Today, I spent cleaning my files. Gemma, try to get the names of all the families at the clinic when you go in April. With the names you've sent me and the ones I had, plus those at the clinic, we may have a mailing list of close to a hundred. And oh, incidentally, Dr. Solomons and I had a nice chat yesterday. He thinks it would be nice if we could all meet in Chicago at the April clinic to talk over the newsletter idea and to get acquainted. I like the idea, but don't know if we could make it, though maybe . . ."

The idea of meeting my newfound friends sounded great. I would definitely be there, but I doubted if any of the others would come. It was an awfully long trip, and money was scarce for most of us.

With satisfaction, I realized that it had been a good idea to put the first newsletter out prior to the appearance of my second *Redbook* piece. Coupled together, the scheduled clinic and the magazine story were already renewing interest in the management and study of OI. The newsletter, though it was only one typewritten page, seemed to be tangible evidence that people afflicted with "brittle bones" did exist in numbers and, indeed, were very hungry for information and emotional support.

From Barbara, I heard, "Two years have passed since we linked the miles. What a different kind of feeling I have about life today. Very few days pass that I don't stop and thank God for all his blessings. There aren't enough words or paper to write on to thank you for your most needed support. Thank you, dear, dear Gemma!

"We have an appointment with a local doctor. We need a recommendation before we can get Gregg into a hospital. I plan to go armed with my newsletter and the information you have sent us. Thank you again for sending the newsletter. It was what we needed to get us started."

"I'm so pleased with the newsletter," Renee wrote. "So pleased . . . so elated. So much is happening—your article coming, the possible meeting in Chicago. (Oh, I hope we can go!) I find it hard to concentrate on anything until I sit down to write to you and Becky."

"I can hardly wait for the March issue of *Redbook*!" came from Midge. "If the newsletter is a hint of the article, it'll be great. It's all I can think of!"

If I had not already been filled with enthusiasm about the newsletter and the article, these letters would certainly have provided the spark to ignite it. Waiting for "Epilogue" to be published was so unlike the time when Dick and I had waited with guarded optimism for my first story to appear. This time, we didn't wait alone. We were being lavished with joyous expectation by a circle of loyal friends. I prayed that I wouldn't let them down.

Late one evening in early February, I learned that the March issue had finally hit the newsstands. Phoning from California, her voice choked with tears, a mother told me, "I just read 'Epilogue to a Dream' in *Redbook* magazine. I couldn't believe it at first, so I read it again and again. I have a small son with osteogenesis imperfecta, and until now, I had never heard of anyone else with the same problem. Your article is an answer to our prayers."

Because of the interest the first article had generated, I expected a respectable response from the follow-up. Instead, I was literally buried by an avalanche. My quiet, contented days became a steady confusion of letters and phone calls. They came from the most remote places, from the desolate, the astonished, the cynical, the happy, the tearful, and the rejoicing.

His voice husky with emotion, a young man from Louisiana said, "Mrs. Geisman, our doctor is outraged at you and *Redbook* for giving us hope for our little boy. But I wanted to tell you how happy *we* are. Actually, what I really wanted to do was to be able to talk with someone who still believes in hope."

The calls came all hours of the day and night. Women were reading the magazine in beauty shops, laundromats, and doctors' offices. One of them said to me, "I was sitting under a hair dryer at the beauty shop, flipping the pages of a magazine, when suddenly the words osteogenesis imperfecta leaped out at me from the page. I did a double take. I thought my eyes were playing tricks on me, so I turned each page over again carefully, hoping to find out that what I had seen was really true. I finally found it on page 89 and read quickly while still under the hair dryer. When the beauty operator came to lift the hood off my head, she asked why I was crying. I told her, 'I was reading a sad story in a magazine, and could I please take it home to finish it?' She gave it to me, and I went home to devour the words over and over again and still, I can't believe it! Since our son was born with OI, this is the first time I've been able to read anything on the subject. I had to call you to make sure you were real, that the story was real."

Another mother recounted a story about a gift from a neighbor. She said, "I've lived on this street for a number of years, and ever since our little boy was born with OI, the other mothers in the neighborhood have stayed away and haven't allowed their children to play with Matt. I've always told myself that I understood why when I really didn't. This morning, my doorbell rang, and when I answered it, I found a woman about my age standing there whom I recognized as a neighbor. She had tears in her eyes and a magazine in her hands. She said, 'I've brought you something. Can I come in?' I invited her in and took the magazine she extended to me. She opened it for me to a marked page and said, 'Go ahead, read it.' I read, and as I did, the whole glorious, wonderful thing came to me. Someone had written with hope about OI, and this woman had brought it to me as a gift. I went to her and embraced her. 'I've wanted to be your friend for a long time,' she said. 'But you always seemed sadly preoccupied with your little boy, I didn't know how to approach you. Then I read this story and knew it was what I needed to open the door without seeming rude or curious about Matt.' Because of your article," the mother recounting the story said, "I have a new friend. I wanted to call to tell you how happy you've made me."

For me, it was a bittersweet time. I had never been so happy, yet so sad. For every joyful letter and phone call, there were two of anguish and tears.

A mother sent a photograph of her child for me to diagnose. A frantic father wrote from Mexico for an appointment to bring his OI son to me for examination. Someone had told him that I was an expert on the disorder. A teenage boy asked in a painstakingly written note, "Do you think it's too late for me?"

A young Irish mother, living in Canada, sent me newspaper clippings about her horrifying ordeal of being jailed under suspicion of physically abusing her three children who suffered frequent unexplained fractures. "Imagine our terror!" she wrote. "We loved our children, and we were worried sick about them, and we were being accused of willfully harming them!" Needless to say, the parents had demanded tests and further x-rays, and all three children had ultimately been diagnosed as having osteogenesis imperfecta in varying degrees. Several other letters confirmed that, in cases of milder OI, especially those not diagnosed at birth, suspicions of child abuse were becoming increasingly common. This was a frightening discovery, and one I definitely didn't have the experience or know-how to deal with, so I referred them to Dr. Millar at Shriners.

Other parents, I learned, weren't fortunate enough to have someone like Dr. Millar to turn to. "We've never had much hope for our little boy," one mother wrote. "The doctors never really try to answer our questions. They simply walk away or try to change the subject when we ask them things about OI. If we ask, how can we help our child, or where can we take him for care? they say, 'Nothing can be done. There is no help.'"

Another said, "The other day, I was walking down the hospital corridor with my son's pediatrician, begging him to at least try to find a way to help our child. But all he did was shrug and pull away from me, saying, 'I have better things to do with my time. Please excuse me.'"

Of course, not all doctors were like him. Another parent wrote, "The orthopedist who has treated our son for most of his life is marvelous. He is medically competent, but even more important, he is willing to use every skill and resource at his command. And he is human. He knows that when a small boy says his leg hurts, it hurts regardless of what can or cannot be seen on an x-ray. He knows that in a case of OI, anything is possible, and he is always on the alert."

I was appalled by some of the things I heard and read, heartened by others. Needless to say, the letters made me realize that dialogue among the parents was essential. So much could be learned by sharing experiences. Not only desired, but also very necessary, was better communication with the doctors responsible for the care of our children. It would be a huge challenge, but I envisioned our newsletter becoming our best means of bridging this wide communication gap.

As mixed as the response to the article was, it did not in any way lessen the fun that it brought to my family and me. One evening, one of my brothers and several of my sisters got together with my elderly mother to phone their congratulations. Former teachers, old school chums, and friends not heard from in years wrote delighted notes of recognition. Newspapers from neighboring cities and towns called for interviews. A TV station invited me to appear on a popular talk show, and *Redbook*'s public relations staff phoned often to follow up on the local and national reaction.

Our children had an immediate rise in stock and prestige at school, and they capitalized shamelessly. Cathy's friends, who usually didn't give me a second glance, now looked at me with admiration. And when I made my TV debut, Cindy and Dickie were given special permission to watch during classes at their usually strict parochial school.

Even though Mike often bragged about being the sole inspiration for all that was happening, he now seemed quieter, more thoughtful than usual. One day, I looked up from my desk where I was answering letters, and I saw him in the doorway quietly watching me.

"What's on your mind?" I asked.

He hesitated, then shrugged. "Nothing."

I prodded. "Things are better for us now, aren't they?"

"Yes, but . . ." he stammered.

"But what?"

"One of my friends told me you said you hated me in your first magazine story," he blurted.

My heart jumped in my throat. Tears filled my eyes.

Before I could answer, he quickly added, "I told him he was wrong, that it was the bone disease you hated, not me!"

"That's what I tried to say, that I hated OI, but loved you. Remember, we talked about it before I would let the magazine publish it?"

Barely above a whisper, he confided, "I hate OI too. I think I told you that then. And yeah, things are better now that we know those other mothers and their kids and the doctors trying to help us."

"Would you like to read both of the *Redbook* articles now? Then we could talk about them again?"

"Naw," he said, grinning and waving me away as he had done two years earlier. "Whatever you said in them is okay with me. It couldn't be that bad. Look at all the good stuff that's happening because of them."

I don't know if Mike ever read the *Redbook* stories. I suspect he might have done so on the sly. But I don't recall him ever mentioning them again. And though we heatedly debated many controversial topics as he grew older and bolder, we never again spoke of doubts concerning our love for each other.

Chapter Sixteen

The frequent letters from our mothers' group served as a delightful antidote to the heartbreak letters that were arriving daily. Everyone mentioned in my article was caught up in a dizzying whirl of activity and publicity that had swelled from one small ripple to an ever-growing circle that now included doctors and hospitals as well as parents and patients.

Renee's thoughts never failed to brighten. "I have received so many of your letters lately, and the lift to your spirits is evident in all of them," she remarked in one of her letters. "I have read so many times the article, and each time, I am touched—brought to tears—at the manner in which it is able to get to the heart of the subject and make one live each moment, each thought, and know the joys and sorrows.

"I have received phone calls from parents of OI children in this area and one visit from the parents of a three-year-old girl. It seems everyone is starved for some kind of communication. I've also discovered what a rare experience it is to be able to talk openly to others who know about OI.

"In a sense, spring has come and gone here in Alabama, but it was nice while it lasted. The budding trees, bright yellow daffodils, and delicate pink tulips still add their touch of color to the cold stormy day and remind us of the three days of warm sun we had prior to the cold front. I couldn't help but compare the busyness of the children during the warm sunny days to our own eagerness to share our good news about the research with each other and the rest of the world. The children wanted to make the most of the sunshine for it had been a long time since they'd enjoyed such loveliness and warmth, and we wanted to share our good news with all, for it had been a long time since we'd had such good news. I think that, in this thought, there is a lesson for us. There will be other sunny days."

"We've been to Shriners Hospital!" Barbara cheerfully announced. "The trip to the Massachusetts Unit is 136 miles one way, and we had to get up at 4:00 a.m., but the day was beautiful in every way. The weather was great. We didn't get lost. But most important of all, Gregg was placed on their waiting list!

"The chief surgeon knows Dr. Millar and is familiar with the research program going on at the Chicago Unit. We told him that we had applied with Dr. Solomons for the magnesium oxide treatment through our private physician, and he seemed quite pleased.

"There are nine doctors on the staff there, and we saw all but one. Gregg was quite impressed with the men in green coats, but he was also a little tense. Poor darling, he's been so sheltered, and he has had so little medical attention. I tried to prepare him for the visit as best I could, but I'm afraid the x-ray machine still looked like a monster to him!

"There are sixty beds at this hospital, and the waiting list is long. When Gregg is admitted, it will be for an overall examination to determine his general physical condition and to decide whether he is strong enough to undergo surgery. We aren't fooling ourselves into thinking that we can do the impossible for him. If they can help him, we'll be happy. But if they can't, at least we will have tried.

"The new x-rays showed no change since birth. After studying them, the chief surgeon told us that Gregg would never walk, but then we've always known this. There is a possibility that they can straighten his arms and teach him to sit erect. This is all we're asking.

"It has been a long day, and I'm happily exhausted. I wanted to take time out to say thanks, for without your support, my outlook on life would be altogether different. You were with us today in that waiting room, each and everyone of you."

From Midge, I heard, "So much is happening—so many wonderful things since the article. Yesterday, our insurance man came in as I was finishing your last letter, and I was just splitting at the seams to talk to someone about it, so I'm afraid I took advantage of the first person who came along and really talked my heart out. When he left, he said he was going right out to buy the magazine. At noon, Mark and I walked to a neighbor's so I could talk some more. It was a marvelous day in every way. Hearing from you, then from Barb a letter saying they were finally getting help for Gregg, makes me want to go around singing all the time!"

Becky asked, "Will life ever be the same again? I am literally swamped with mail and phone calls, so I know what you must be experiencing, Gemma. I had no inkling this was going to happen, but oh, how I prayed! Somehow, I have always felt that there were many children with OI out there who needed help, but there simply had to be more cases than the few we knew about, but I didn't realize there could be so many! Now that we know there are, we must keep this thing going. I think we've finally found the right combination—the right people at the right time—and it's working. It's going to keep working. I know it. I can feel it!"

The ingredients for an attack against OI seemed right to me too. Dr. Solomons, Dr. Millar, and Shriners Hospital were also being flooded with letters; and with commendable spirit, they immediately made up an application and form letter to handle the influx. Meanwhile, our group of mothers was working overtime acknowledging every phone call and letter with a copy of the newsletter and a personal message of hope. Our combined efforts quickly reaped amazing results.

Within a matter of weeks, Becky and I noticed a definite pattern emerging. On the West Coast, the magazine had come out nearly a week ahead of other areas. Therefore, our first inquiries had come flooding in from California. Typically, almost everyone who wrote knew of only one, or of no others, with the disorder. Yet as I studied a California map, I noticed that most of the early inquiries had come from the San Francisco area, followed by Los Angeles, then San Diego.

Interested in this new development, I wrote to Becky and asked whether she had noticed the same thing. She assured me that she had. Moreover, she had asked Charles to install a huge wall map in her cubicle office so she could follow the emerging pattern. With small identifying pins—red for girls and blue for boys—she marked the geographical location of every family we heard from.

Soon, we were using file cards to keep track of the growing list of families and the pertinent medical information they were sending. With a package of duplicate cards I was mailing to Becky, I casually mentioned in a note that we had enough names in California to start some kind of organization or support group. That's all she needed. She wrote back, "That's a great idea!"

As the magazine appeared in the mail and newsstands in other sections of the country, the pattern repeated itself, particularly around heavily populated areas. In New York, Pennsylvania, and Illinois, OI families began to meet informally with hopes of organizing chapters. Without us realizing it, the seeds had germinated and begun to sprout.

By mid-April, our people from Northern California had met, formed a chapter based on hopes and dreams rather than guidelines, and elected officers. A Los Angeles group was in the process of forming, and in San Diego, a small group of families was planning to band together.

Sheer enthusiasm got us through those exciting, yet complex days. People everywhere were looking to us for structure when we had none. For over four hundred years, no knowledge about OI, other than rare mentions in medical textbooks, had been available. Now families and even doctors were seeking advice from us! Our own personal experiences with OI was all we had, so we shared those. There had never been much medical or community support for most of us, but the emotional support we were now getting from one another was priceless. So we shared that too the best we could.

The Chicago meeting, originally meant to be a pleasant rendezvous, now became a means—a target date, so to speak—of getting together to figure out where all this activity was leading us. The newly formed groups expected us to set guidelines and objectives, then oversee their progress. Taking on this leadership role was definitely something we needed to discuss, and the Chicago meeting seemed the appropriate time and place to do so.

In the meantime, Dr. Solomons was having challenges of his own with the financial aspects of his research. Funded by Shriners, Colorado General, and with the aid of a research grant from the National Institutes of Health, his work had progressed well. But now, he was faced with the possible cancellation of government funds due to the administration's sharp cutbacks at this very crucial time when countless families with OI children were contacting him for help. Hoping that the increased number of patients to study would give his grant higher priority with the politicians, he urged us to write to our congressmen with the request that his grant be renewed.

Working at a feverish pace, we put a letter out to our members asking them to write to their Washington representatives. Within a matter of days, President and Mrs. Nixon, the National Institutes of Health, and nearly every politician in Washington had heard about OI and Dr. Solomons's research. For many of them, the photos of children with OI was their first encounter with the disorder, and as is often the case, the pictures had shaken them up. Letters signed with prominent signatures arrived daily with promises and assurances that everything possible would be done to ensure the renewal of Dr. Solomons's grant. Naively, we believed them and expected them to follow through. Most did not.

"Poor Dr. Solomons!" Becky wrote after it was all over. "I think he would like to go hide on a quiet tropical isle with his family for about a month! His phone rings constantly with pleas for help. I can't imagine what would happen if his grant was dropped. So many are counting on him. I think he's beginning to feel the weight of the responsibility."

At about the same time, I too would have gladly escaped to a tropical isle with Dick and the children. People were writing and calling at all hours, asking, "We've written to our congressmen, now what?" I must confess that it was at that point that I began using the Chicago meeting as a put off by telling those who asked that we were having a meeting in Chicago in April to determine our next move. "Please be patient," I told them. "More details about the meeting will follow in our newsletter."

Those few words meant to appease and to buy us time had entirely different results. Now the questions being asked were whether they could come to Chicago for the meeting and where and what time was the meeting being held. Who was in charge of reservations, and what topics did we have on the agenda?

The agenda? What agenda?

Confused, I contacted Becky and asked, "Hey, what's going on?"

In her calm, understated manner, she replied. "Now, Gemma, we have to get hold of ourselves and get something ready . . . some program or something. These people are counting on us."

"I plan to bring the information I've accumulated—the letters and the names and addresses of those who want to form state associations," I mumbled. "But, Becky, I've never organized the kind of meeting they expect!"

"I'm bringing my card file, and I hope to add to it by getting as many families as I can to sign up. A man with OI from New Jersey has a public relations firm. He's promised to come and help us. There's also a couple from Georgia interested in coming. They said they'd look into the legal aspects of this thing for us, if we wanted them to. Others have also indicated interest," she continued, breathless with excitement.

"You know that I planned to have this get-together in our motel rooms, don't you? Of course, that'll be out of the question with so large a group."

But there was no dissuading Becky. "I'll see if Dr. Solomons will mention to Dr. Millar that we're coming. Maybe they'll let us have one of the meeting rooms at the hospital. Listen, Gemma, you take care of the reservations and keep telling everyone about the meeting. I'll take care of the rest. Okay?"

A few days later, we received notice that Mike was to be admitted to Shriners for more surgery the following week. I hadn't counted on an extra trip to Chicago and another bout of surgery for Mike, so this particular letter hit hard. Immersed in hope, we had pushed aside the grim realities of the limitations of surgery, the restrictions of casts, and the loneliness brought on by the long separations.

To compensate for what couldn't be avoided, I filled Mike's remaining days at home with special attention by cooking his favorite foods and by giving him an early birthday party. School chums, neighborhood pals, and family members came bearing gifts of records, books, and games. It was fun while it lasted, but when all was said and done, and Mike had been admitted to the hospital, the usual feeling of helplessness and emptiness permeated our hearts.

Returning home, I plunged with renewed determination into the mountain of mail and the increasing number of details that needed attention. I answered all inquiries about the meeting; and with the help of Frances Dubowski, my friend, the OI clinic nurse at Shriners, motel accommodations were found, and reservations made for all who wanted to come. From Dr. Millar, I learned that the hospital's finest meeting room would be at our disposal.

During an evening phone call just days before the meeting, Renee advised me that Becky's agenda called for a welcoming speech from me in which I would discuss plans for a national osteogenesis imperfecta association.

"Me! Give a welcoming address! No way!" I shrieked. "I'll die on the spot. No, I can't do it! I won't!" Just thinking of making a speech was enough to nauseate me and make my knees go weak.

Becky had not only given me a speech assignment, she was advertising it as well. I learned about that from a South Dakota mother who phoned and said, "Becky Keller told me that you're speaking at the Chicago meeting. Could you tell me what the arrangements are? We wouldn't want to miss it!"

To myself, I moaned, *Why is Becky doing this to me?* Yet from within my being, another voice prompted me to be nice to the lady and invite her to attend. And as the day of the meeting grew nearer, that same inner voice constantly arranged and revised in my mind the words I would speak in Chicago.

From this constant sorting out of words, it became obvious that the overwhelming needs were for emotional support and better medical intervention and more basic research and current information about osteogenesis imperfecta. These were more than enough reasons to forge ahead with plans for a national nonprofit organization for OI. The manner by which these objectives would be pursued was all that remained unclear. For this, we would have to rely on the help of others.

Long before the day of the meeting, I knew I was fully committed and determined to give my speech even though I dreaded that doing so might bring about an acute episode of stage fright—a fear that *did* materialize on the fateful day but was quickly covered up with the help and sustenance of those who stood beside me.

Chapter Seventeen

Jokingly, I had told Becky to wear a carnation in her lapel so I would know her when finally we met since she was the only one who hadn't sent a photograph. We were to meet at Shriners Hospital as soon as the doors opened; and as Dick and I drove through endless lines of grinding and screeching Chicago traffic, I tried to imagine what this woman, who had become one of my closest friends, would be like. Having shared so much with each other in our letters, I felt confident that we would have the same warm relationship up close and personal.

To divert my attention from the anxiety I felt about having to make a speech in front of a crowd, I played silent games as we rode. First, I watched the pale yellow sun peeking around the corners of drab tall buildings, saw it dance briefly on the windshield, then disappear again behind sooty, towering skyscrapers. Then I searched the faces of the people zooming past in their cars to see if I could catch someone smiling. *Finding a happy face in Chicago's early-morning commuter traffic would be a good omen*, I told myself. But no matter what sort of diversion I chose, nothing seemed able to distract my mind from the chore at hand, nor would it stop the pounding of my heart or the lurching sensation in my stomach.

The door to the familiar clinic room swung open at Dick's effortless touch, and suddenly, we were in the midst of a noisy crowd. Never before had we seen this room so full and so loud with sounds of joy and laughter.

Suddenly, a spell of dizziness washed over me, and I swayed. Dick steadied me and, looking worried, asked, "Are you all right?"

I laughed. "I'm a little giddy from all the excitement, I guess!"

Scanning the room quickly, I spotted three elfin-faced little boys clustered together, talking and laughing in thin, chiming voices; and I knew instantly, from having seen their photos, that they were Mark, Donny, and Doug. Pulling away from Dick, I hurried over to them.

Mark Peck greeted me with merry, sparkling eyes and, as if he'd known me all his life, said, "Hi, Mrs. Geisman! When's Mike coming out of the ward? When can we see him?"

Doug looked me over with dark, somber eyes, and Donny smiled shyly as he gave me a businesslike appraisal.

"Mike will be discharged after the clinic is over, then all you guys can get acquainted at the motel," I told them. For Mark, who had brought his tricycle, I added, "But mind you, there won't be any tricycle races. Mike will be in a great big cast."

They all groaned at the mention of the word *cast*, then went back to their chatter as I moved away to find their mothers.

Looking expectantly into the crowd, my eyes met those of a delicate-looking young woman, wearing a bright yellow dress. "Is it you, Renee?" I asked.

We hugged warmly; then backing away, she laughed. "You are Gemma, aren't you?" I nodded, and she smiled as she shook herself and said, "I still can't believe this is happening. I keep thinking I'm going to wake up and discover that it's all been a dream."

"It does seem unreal," I agreed. "It's all happening so fast. I feel like I'm on a roller-coaster ride, afraid to stay on but too late to get off."

Grinning, she grabbed my hand. "The ride won't be as bumpy if we hold on to each other," she said. "You haven't met Midge and Becky yet, have you? You'll love them both. Becky and I were together at the motel last night, and this morning, Don and the boys and I had breakfast with Midge, Dewey, and Mark." She stretched her neck to search above the crowd. "They're around here somewhere," she continued. "You wait here. I'll go find them for you."

As I watched Renee weave her way across the room, I felt a tap on my shoulder and turned around. Behind me was a slim woman with short curly brown hair. Her face was so much like Mark's—the same bright-eyed look, the same turned-up smile. I knew right away that it had to be Midge.

"Gemma!" she exclaimed, her arms reaching out, and like old friends, we embraced. "We're all here together, finally, just as we planned," she said, sighing with satisfaction.

"Oh Midge, it's so good to see you at last! I've already met Mark. He's a wonderful boy."

She beamed. "He is, isn't he?" Then pulling at my hand, she said, "Come and meet Dewey. And of course, I want to meet Dick . . . and Mike, when he's released from the ward. Mark is very anxious to meet his buddy."

Sweet, loving, talkative Midge, I thought to myself as I followed behind her. She too was exactly the way I had imagined her to be.

As Midge and I pushed our way through the crowd, my arm brushed against someone, and a wonderful sense of familiarity washed over me. I turned to look over my shoulder as Midge walked on and saw a tanned-looking tall woman with light brown hair pulled away from a high forehead, looking straight at me. A spark of recognition ignited her expressive dark eyes. At the same moment, I realized that the woman wearing slacks and a Western-style blouse had to be Becky from Cactus Patch Ranch.

For a brief suspended moment, neither one of us spoke as we examined each other's faces to see if we were truly what we had hoped to be to each other. Her eyes brimming with unshed tears, she reached for my hands and held them in her strong grasp. "Well, Gemma, here we are," she said, her voice thick with emotion. "We've come a long way, you and I."

"Yes, we have," I murmured, remembering the long, lonely years before we'd known each other.

Giving me another quick hug, she said, "We'll talk loads later, okay? Right now, there's so much to do."

At that moment, I wanted nothing more than to gather my newfound friends around me for a pleasant day of getting acquainted, but Becky was right; there was so little time and so much to do. Going to the reception window, I advised the staff that everyone had arrived. They, in turn, informed me that we had the hospital administrator's permission to speak to everyone at the clinic and gather whatever information they were willing to give us. Nurse Frances Dubowski would help us if we had any questions. After the clinic examinations were over, Drs. Millar and Solomons would address the audience, then the floor would be ours.

Becky winked at me at the mention of the floor being ours. "You'll do all right," she said. "I have all the faith in the world in you. Now come, there are people I want you to meet."

First, she introduced me to Arlys Norling (the South Dakota mother who had phoned me about the meeting), her husband, and their son, Doug. Next, she led me to a group of men seated together. To my relief, I found Dick, whom I had abandoned at the door, engaged in earnest conversation with them. Shamefaced, I apologized to my husband and began to make introductions, but they waved me off saying that they had already taken the liberty of introducing themselves. Midge and Renee, who had rejoined us, introduced me to their husbands. Dewey Peck and Dick, I soon discovered, had a lot in common and were even now trading camping and fishing stories.

Because Becky's husband, Charles, hadn't been able to get away; good-looking Joe had accompanied his mother and little brother. He too sat with the men. Also in the group was a lanky, soft-spoken, kindly looking man who introduced himself as Roy Burdette, the father of Brooks, his son with OI, from Hogansville, Georgia. With him was a friendly big bear of a man, his brother-in-law, Thad Aycock. Both appeared to have come prepared to work.

A dark, handsome man wearing a navy blue blazer with an airline emblem on the breast pocket had flown in from California for the meeting. Bob Lutzinger was the father of little Jennifer who had OI. The PR man from New Jersey that Becky had mentioned to me was also there. George Selvin had a milder form of OI, and though he was of short stature and could walk, he had a severe hearing problem. Nevertheless, he owned and operated a successful public relations firm that he was willing to put at our disposal.

The responsibilities that our small group of mothers had shouldered for so long were about to shift to some of these other willing and more experienced volunteers. Gratefully, I thanked them for coming and told them about the day's agenda. All agreed that we needed to sit down together to map out a plan for a national organization. To do that, a lot would have to be accomplished before the day was done.

While the children and their parents were being tested and examined, we set up a table in the back corner of the room and invited those who were waiting to come back to talk to us about their experiences and give us their thoughts about forming a national organization. Additionally, we asked that each family fill out a registry card that would include their OI family history, number of fractures, types of surgery, and other pertinent medical information. At first, some of them appeared shy about divulging this kind of information, but with Midge, Renee, Becky, and I moving among them, they soon came around. Some of them who knew me from previous clinics told me that they had enjoyed the *Redbook* story about their research experience and would be happy to help with a national organization. Others discussed their problems and asked for advice and solutions. Being asked for help was a challenging experience. But it sure felt good to be able to say with some conviction that working together, we *would* find the answers.

The exhilaration and confidence I felt was not to last long, however. While circulating around the room, I was about to approach a group of women seated together when I overheard one of them telling the others, "When I read that woman's first article, I was shocked and disgusted. I couldn't even finish it! How could a mother be so heartless and cruel? It was inhuman of her to write what she did!"

Cringing, I moved away from them on legs that had turned to mush. The pain and heartbreak of those long-ago and nearly forgotten years came surging back. Maybe this woman was right. Maybe I shouldn't have been so frank about my loathsome, mixed feelings. As I floundered about in a quandary, I heard the sound of a familiar voice responding.

It was Midge speaking. "Many parents of OI children have feelings like Gemma's," she said, her voice shaking. "But only a few are brave enough to admit they have them and then do something about them. It's those who can't admit that problems exist that I pity," she added as she walked away, her head held high. The woman who had spoken stared at Midge in disbelief. Midge gave me a quick, compassionate glance; and at that moment, I knew that under the gay, garrulous exterior was a Midge who had suffered a great deal.

Minutes later, a group of doctors appeared in the room. Of those present, I knew only Dr. Millar, Dr. Solomons, and some of the residents. The others, we learned later, had heard about the research from parents who had read my article and, because of their interest in the disorder, had come to observe. Among them was Dr. James Albright, visiting from Yale, as well as specialists from the Hospital for Special Surgery at Cornell. Drs. Millar and Solomons spoke briefly; then with a flourish and a smile, Dr. Millar said, "Now I give the floor to Mrs. Geisman, who will speak to you about a national organization for osteogenesis imperfecta."

Still shaken by the condemning words I had just overheard and with the knowledge that eminent doctors were waiting to hear from me, I rose from my chair. *Dear god, what am I doing here?* my mind screamed. *I'm not the right person for this!*

Realizing my panic, Becky rose from her seat and accompanied me to the front of the room. Without a word, Midge and Renee followed. I watched George Selvin draw his chair closer so he could hear, saw Don Gardner, Roy Burdette, and Thad Aycock turn on their tape recorders. Anxiously, I searched for Dick among the crowd of intent faces focused on me and found him. He smiled an encouraging smile that said, "Go on. You can do it." Reassured, I began to speak.

At first, the words I had rehearsed came easily. Then without warning, the room began to sway, and suddenly, I was caught up in a terrifying whirlpool of spinning faces. Briefly, I saw an edge of darkness and thought, *I'm going to faint in front of all these people!*

Desperately, I drew a deep breath, backed up against the reception window, and clutched the ledge behind my back. In the maze of churning faces, I saw Midge, Becky, and Renee back up with me, lifting me up from the depths with their support. Slowly, the room stilled itself, and to my astonishment, I found that I hadn't stopped talking during my dizzying episode. Amazingly, the words I'd rehearsed about our hopes and dreams for a national organization remained clear and strong and full of conviction. I decided then and there that this was definitely a very good time to wrap things up. My three loyal cohorts expressed briefly their hopes that everyone present would join in the fight against OI, then quickly adjourned the program. As for me, I made a mental note to never ever speak publicly again. How could I have foreseen that this harrowing encounter with stage fright was not about to be my last?

Chapter Eighteen

At noon, with Mike happily in tow, we drove to the motel where everyone was staying. No doubt, our group must have seemed like a strange-looking bunch to the other guests. Mike sat in a semireclining position in his wheelchair, his casted leg propped up on the only thing we could find—an empty ice bucket turned upside down on his footrest. Doug Keller, also sporting a small cast on one leg, bopped merrily on his little bottom. Donny Gardner scuffled about in a football crouch with hands propped on his knees, and because he knew I spoke the language, Mark Peck spouted French phrases he'd learned at school as he pedaled his blue tricycle from room to room. Our excitement being together made us oblivious to any curious glances. None of that mattered now. Being together was what counted.

As we ate a picnic lunch from a nearby restaurant, our boys joked with one another like life-long friends while their fathers discussed fishing and baseball and their mothers talked about the morning's upsets and successes. Satisfied that we had survived the stage fright episode, the swipes, the compliments, and the praises with equal dignity, we decided that the afternoon session should definitely be easier.

Leaving the children and their fathers at the motel after lunch, Becky, Renee, Midge, and I returned to Shriners where we were ushered, like dignitaries, into an impressive-looking meeting room. Slightly overwhelmed by the grand boardroom, we sat down, placed our stacks of papers on the table in front of us, and waited in silence. Gathered around the long polished table were eight quiet, but very determined-looking people.

It was Roy Burdette who finally broke the ice. His features intense with years of frustration, he said, "For so long, we've been told that nothing could be done, and now we find that there is something we can do after all. I know I'm going to do everything in my power to see that this organization gets going. I *have* to be part of this undertaking."

Knowing that we would need this kind of resolve to succeed, I applauded him silently and mentally placed his name on the nomination list for president. Sitting back, I waited to hear from the other newcomers. Having been preoccupied for so long with the many problems afflicting the families who had written or phoned me, I feared I would be more emotional than objective. Looking fatigued, Becky too remained silent.

Little by little, those who sat around the table began to speak about their experiences with OI—their suppressed hopes, their long-festering disappointments, their sadness, and their frustrations. A powerhouse of sentiments was uncorked, hearts emptied, and finally came the resolution to do everything possible so no one would ever again have to cope with osteogenesis imperfecta alone and without hope.

"Gemma, I'm sure you realize that the purposes you defined in your talk this morning were quite specific," Bob Lutzinger said. "I think we should adopt them for our organization then work around them. That is, if everyone is agreeable."

The purposes I had mentioned were threefold—to offer emotional support to affected families, to educate them and the public about OI, and to encourage and support OI research.

"I have been doing a lot of thinking about purposes," Roy said, "and I'm impressed that we have all come up with the same ideas without consulting each other. It shows that we share the same thoughts. I'm in agreement that the fore-mentioned purposes should stand as the official mission of our organization."

Clearly, we were all aware of the needs, so the purposes of our proposed nonprofit organization were quickly agreed upon.

Much discussion concerning a suitable name followed. Though we tried many combinations, we always came back to the Osteogenesis Imperfecta Foundation since we all agreed that the name should clearly spell out who we were and what we intended to do. But as we were well aware, a group using that name had formed in Texas a dozen or so years before. George Selvin suggested that we locate and merge with the Texas group. Becky and I quickly voiced our opposition, stating that the organization had been contacted by both of us and many others without ever a response. It turned out that some of the others seated around the table had experienced the same results. By not responding to simple requests for information, we felt that the first OI Foundation had been delinquent and, therefore, agreed not to align ourselves with them, even if there was a possibility that they still existed.

Someone—I think it was Roy—said, "If one of our purposes is to acquaint the public with osteogenesis imperfecta, then my suggestion is that we incorporate the name of the disorder into the name of the organization somehow. After all, if the public can learn to say *cystic fibrosis*, *cerebral palsy*, and Englebert Humperdinck, they can learn to say osteogenesis imperfecta as well. Only by saying it often and by exposing the public to it can we hope to educate them about it. If we try to camouflage our purposes under some other title, then we are failing at the outset."

The feeling was unanimous, and after further deliberation, it was decided that a search would be made; and if it did not in any way infringe upon the rights of the former foundation, the organization we were incorporating would be known as the Osteogenesis Imperfecta Foundation Inc.

Roy accepted the responsibility of handling the legalities of incorporating a tax-exempt, nonprofit organization, and we all breathed a sigh of relief. Those present were designated charter members of the first board of directors, and I was assigned to seek additional board members from the Shriner and *Redbook* organizations.

Satisfied with what had been accomplished, we closed the meeting and said good-bye to Bob Lutzinger, who was scheduled to fly back to California. We'd barely had time to get to know him, and he was gone—gone with the promise to do all he could to develop and oversee the foundation chapters in California. Art and Arlys Norling departed for their home in South Dakota with a pledge to do all they could. Saying that he'd return the next morning to help us tie up the loose ends, Roy left to spend the night with his relatives, and the rest of us returned to the motel. Once there, box lunches were ordered, sent to our rooms; and in a festive mood, we told our husbands what had been accomplished.

Becky and her children, the Gardners, and George Selvin had early-afternoon flights the next day, and the Pecks had to be on the road early in the morning. Our time together was growing short, and still, we mothers hadn't shared any private time together. Only a few evening hours remained, so we agreed to rendezvous in Becky's room as soon as our tired boys had been put to bed. We'd barely settled in when we were summoned back to my room to meet with new visitors. An attractive couple from a nearby town in Illinois had come to tell us about a soon-to-be published book about their experiences raising Roxie, their teenage daughter with OI.

Though they informed us that they had just become grandparents, John and Beverly Plummer had a youngish Bohemian look about them. Both wore cotton shirts and flared jeans. A shaggy, boyish haircut framed Beverly's expressive face, and John was tall and had blond, curly-haired good looks. They had come to meet with us because the publisher of Beverly's forthcoming book *Give Every Day a Chance* had heard about Dr. Solomons's research and wanted her to mention it in the epilogue she was preparing for her book. Meeting another mother willing to share her experiences with the rest of the world was a nice footnote to an already wonderful day.

George Selvin was more than impressed with Beverly's accomplishment, and he suggested that she join our efforts since she would have the perfect opportunity to publicize the start of the foundation while promoting her book. Beverly graciously declined involvement in the organizational work but promised to mention the foundation in her epilogue.

Determined to find every resource he could for us, George also suggested, after the Plummers had gone, that we attempt to contact Rosarie Geiger, a Pennsylvania woman who had kept a national registry of OI patients for an interested physician who ran a clinic at Johns Hopkins. It would be good business, he advised, to obtain this national registry of OI patients and add it to our own fast-growing list. We agreed with him that it would indeed eliminate a lot of work for us and enable us to reach a larger number of families. Armed with the information he provided us, we attempted to phone Mrs. Geiger and were told that she was not at home, but that she would most certainly want to return our call that same evening.

Several hours passed without a return call. Excusing himself, George Selvin retired for the night. Regretfully, Midge and Dewey did the same since they had a long ride ahead of them the next morning. Appearing totally wiped out and sounding apologetic, Becky also begged off. "I didn't get a wink of sleep last night," she said. "Maybe I should try getting some tonight."

"Go on, get some sleep," Renee urged. "I'll stay with Gemma until the call comes."

Knowing that we wanted to talk, Dick turned his attention to the late news on TV, and Renee and I sat on the other side of the room speaking quietly for hours about our separate lives and about the hopes and dreams we had for our fledgling organization.

Our phone call to Mrs. Geiger was never returned. In the early-morning hours, Renee tiptoed away to her room. It seemed I had just fallen asleep when Mike and Dick were shaking me awake to tell me that everyone was up and getting ready to meet for breakfast.

We ate with the Pecks; then after everyone else had told them good-bye, we returned to their room with them to visit while they packed. On motel notepaper, Midge and I wrote a hurried letter to Barbara St. Amour to tell her about the meeting. We wanted her to be a part of it in this small way since she hadn't been able to attend. Then our two families said good-bye, along with a promise to get together again real soon.

Determined to have some time with Becky, I hurried to her room only to find her gone. Joe said she'd been on her way to see me when she'd run into Roy Burdette and George Selvin, who were headed for the Gardner's quarters for a wrap-up session.

Becky shrugged helplessly when she saw me. It was apparent that she too was getting frustrated by our inability to spend personal time together. Understanding perfectly how she was feeling, I sat next to her on the edge of the bed and held her hand. The men were already discussing the legalities and fine points of the previous day's business, and Renee was trying to write it down for the record. Everything sounded so complicated. I thought, *Thank goodness for Roy Burdette!* We could never have done this without him!

Evidently, everyone else felt as I did. Before adjourning, we unanimously agreed to nominate Roy for the position of president. Bob Lutzinger was nominated vice president; Renee, treasurer; and Becky, secretary. With George Selvin's help, I would develop literature, edit the newsletter, and remain as spokesperson for the foundation.

As they boarded the limousine that would take them to the airport, George Selvin and Roy Burdette reaffirmed their commitments with firm handshakes. Don Gardner told us good-bye and herded the children into the waiting vehicle. Clinging together, tears intermingling, Becky, Renee, and I said good-bye.

Mike, Dick, and I remained in the motel parking lot until the limousine entered the busy thruway and meshed in with the flow of speeding automobiles.

"Mom, can we please go home now?" Mike pleaded.

"Yes, let's go home. We have lots of work to do if we're going to get this organization going," I replied, and as I spoke, I thought I heard my son and husband collectively breathe a loud sigh that sounded like "Whatever are we in for now?"

Chapter Nineteen

The end of the school year was near, and Mike had been assigned to give an oral presentation over his telephone hookup for his junior high speech class.

"Dress up in your best duds, just like you would if you were speaking in front of them," I told him, repeating the advice I had read about practicing speeches. I'd been devouring books on public speaking ever since my nearly disastrous experience in Chicago.

"Aw, Mom," he protested. "It won't make any difference. They can't see me."

"C'mon, try it!" I pleaded.

"Well, all right," he said, giving in to humor me.

His best pants wouldn't fit over his bulky cast, so he put on his favorite shirt, neatly brushed his hair, and waited nervously for the teacher to call on him.

When finally she did, I held down the button on the intercom so his classmates could hear him, and he began to speak. One minute, he was eloquent, the next humorous. Though we couldn't hear the reaction with the button pushed down, I was certain that his classmates had to be laughing and applauding. When his short, but inspiring, presentation ended, I let go of the button, expecting to hear a loud clamor. But the only sound was silence. Not understanding, I buzzed the teacher.

Sounding sheepish, she said, "I'm sorry, Mike, but we ran out of time in the middle of your presentation, and the class had to be dismissed."

Disgusted, he asked, "You mean I was talking to an empty classroom?"

"It was an A+ speech," the teacher said to console him. "I'm sorry the class didn't get to hear it all."

Letting go of the button that connected him with the teacher, he turned to face me, and I saw that even though his lower lip was trembling a bit, the rest of his face had taken on the stony look that he hid behind when he was hurting. "I wasn't any good, was I? She's giving me an A+ because she feels sorry for me," he sneered, and nothing I could say would convince him otherwise.

Furious at myself and the teacher for not having anticipated such an occurrence, I left Mike's room and went directly to the phone to suggest to her that we had both erred and could never ever let this happen again. Also, I wanted to share with her how Mike had prepared and practiced for his speech, had dressed especially for the occasion, only to be demoralized by the outcome. I needed to make her see that Mike was a bright fourteen-year-old eager to participate in the classroom and not just a voice in little brown box that was carried from classroom to classroom and placed on her desk.

Unfortunately, the teacher had gone to lunch. So to calm myself before tackling another discussion of the incident with Mike, I went to my study to work on choosing a name for the foundation newsletter. Earlier that morning, I had written down possibilities along with their definitions on a yellow legal pad, and as I looked at them again, the word *breakthrough* literally jumped off the page. From *Webster's Dictionary*, I had written *breakthrough*—an offensive operation that pierces a defensive system and reaches the unorganized area behind it.

Would we ever, I wondered, be able to mount an offensive strong enough to pierce through the many layers of ignorance and apathy associated with rare disabilities like osteogenesis imperfecta? And if we did, what would we find in the gray, disorganized area beyond? Acceptance and normalcy for our children? More than ever, I wanted and needed to be an important part of the organized force, and I saw the newsletter as *my* means, *my* instrument for breaking down the barriers. Without consulting anyone, I christened the newsletter *Breakthrough* and developed a slogan for it that read, "Don't give them a break, just a chance!" Dick, who draws well, drew up a nameplate for it; then I proudly sent the four-page issue, chockfull of information about OI and the OI Foundation, to Becky, who thoroughly approved and had it mimeographed and mailed in no time.

After reading the newsletter, Roy Burdette wrote me a tactful letter that praised my efforts but strongly advised that he be allowed to review the contents of future issues so they could be approved by the entire executive board prior to publication. He further admonished me to be more careful about making independent decisions, about endorsing individual research projects, and soliciting donations until we had applied for and obtained our tax-exempt status.

Rereading the newsletter, I realized that Roy was right. The newsletter no longer belonged to Becky and me; it was now the official voice of the OI Foundation. If I was to succeed as spokesperson for the organization, I would have to curb my impatience and tether my hopes and work for the good of all. This proved to be a difficult resolve for me to honor. If occasionally I forgot during the weeks that followed, Roy gently reminded me.

From the almost daily memos and letters I received from Roy and his wife, Mildred, a teacher, I came to know them and love them. It didn't take long for those of us involved in the work of the foundation to realize how lucky we'd been to find them. Their son, Brooks, no doubt inspired their sensitivity and dedication—a hard-to-find combination that was exactly what we needed.

Working at a constant pace, they established communication guidelines, set up bylaws, and did all the chores connected with legally establishing a national nonprofit, tax-exempt organization. This they did through endless consultations with members of the board, now comprised of ten members with the addition of *Redbook* editor Sey Chassler and Mike's former orthopedist at Shriners, Dr. Harold A. Sofield. Not one step was taken, no move made, without the approval of the majority.

After school let out in June, Dick and I took the children on a trip through Eastern Canada and the New England states for a long-awaited visit with my family. While there, we did something I'd been wanting to do for a long time. We spent a day in Exeter, New Hampshire, with Barbara and George St. Amour and their family. Meeting Barbara for the first time was the same as my meeting with the others had been that April day in Chicago. It was filled with a mixture of hugs and tears and joys at being together at last.

Looking at Gregg lying flat on his back in a brand-new cart on wheels, his arms and legs bent beyond repair by countless untreated fractures, his growth incredibly stunted, I ached inside for the smiling, freckle-faced kid and his parents. Silently, I vowed to do all I could to see that every child with OI would get the medical treatment needed. Like us, the St. Amours had suffered a lot of needless pain. But it was obvious that they'd also been blessed with much love and courage.

Gregg's and Mike's reactions to each other were unlike the joking and teasing that had gone on among the boys in Chicago. Both remained quiet as they eyed each other, and several times during our visit, Mike tried to whisper to me that he couldn't believe how bad off Gregg was. I had to shush him up for fear Gregg would hear and be hurt. As for Gregg, he seemed in absolute awe of Mike's expert ability to maneuver a wheelchair.

As we were leaving, Barbara told me, "I don't know what I would've done without your letters and those of the others. You have given our lives new meaning." Tears welled in her eyes, and her chin quivered as she spoke. I hugged her warmly, knowing full well that all I could give her was friendship, understanding, and a little bit of hope.

Back home again, I found an enormous stack of mail waiting. There had been a great deal of busyness during my absence. There were both offers of help and pleas for help. From Becky, Renee, and the Burdettes, I read progress reports that said everything was going slow, but well. However, in a letter from George Selvin was something that didn't sound right to me.

Without the approval of the board, he had set up appointments, he wrote, with representatives of the National Foundation (formerly the March of Dimes organization) in New York City because he felt that we would be better off placing ourselves under their wing. He reasoned that because of their experience, they were better equipped to handle the research and to deal with the multifaceted problems of the disorder.

I couldn't believe what I was reading. I didn't want our efforts swallowed up by a mammoth organization that had not shown any appreciable interest in OI. I knew from experience that other than providing occasional braces or wheelchairs, OI had been all but ignored by the major organizations for the disabled. Years earlier, I had asked a representative of one such organization if they could please help Mike, and her answer had been, "I'm sorry, but we help only those for which there is hope." How stinging those words had been! I had never forgotten them.

Was I being close-minded and stubborn to so readily reject George Selvin's efforts to help? Was I clinging to an impossible dream to want an organization devoted exclusively to osteogenesis imperfecta? After all, the National Foundation had wiped out polio and nearly obliterated the measles, and birth defects were high on their research list. Maybe they could do more than we could. They had the facilities and large sums of money at their disposal. We had neither one.w

But could all their money calm a mother's fear of fracturing her baby while changing his diaper? Could it soften the cruel stares often associated with OI? Could it ease the pain, remove the loneliness of living alone with osteogenesis imperfecta? These were some of the things I strongly believed would be better addressed by a smaller, more personalized group.

As news of a possible merger leaked out to the families who had been working to organize OIF around the country, I discovered many who felt as I did. "Don't do it!" was the emphatic cry. "Now that we have the makings of an organization for OI, don't let go. Don't sell us out!"

Amid the dissension and controversy, Becky wrote, "Gemma, if the majority votes to throw in with the National Foundation, you and I will have to find some way of keeping our people together. We can't let them down. Do you think we could handle and finance *Breakthrough* by ourselves if we had to?"

We both knew that we would do what we had to should the need arise. Fortunately, we didn't have to. After exploring the possibility of merging, Roy and the other board members came through. One of the main factors that led to the decision not to join the larger, better-known organization was a report obtained from the National Foundation that showed that pitifully little OI research had been done and that what was planned for the future was too remotely connected with OI to make any kind of impact.

Several days after our proposed foundation's first skirmish with controversy was settled, we took Mike to Shriners to have his cast removed. It was quiet that day at the hospital. The usually busy clinic rooms were deserted, and all that could be heard was an occasional cry and the buzzing sound of a saw coming from the cast room. For some unexplained reason, Mike was in terrible pain that day. Our fear was that he had fractured his uncasted leg. The excruciating pain made him scream whenever we moved him, and when his cast was removed, he cried uncontrollably, which was very unusual for him. Puzzled, Dr. Millar examined him and ordered x-rays taken, but no fractures were detected. Later, while waiting in the clinic room for Mike's pain to subside before heading home, I once again asked myself how a merciful God could allow a little boy to suffer so much pain.

Appropriately, at that moment, Dr. Solomons came breezing in. Seeing us sitting alone in the clinic room, he did a double take. Since this wasn't a regular clinic day, we too were surprised to see him. He had just happened to be between plane flights at O'Hare, he told us, and, on a whim, had decided to drop in. Barely able to contain his enthusiasm, he told us he was returning home after a visit to the first OI clinic at the Hospital for Special Surgery in New York City.

My dark thoughts dissipated quickly as I listened to his ecstatic descriptions of the well-equipped hospital, the interested staff, and the large group of patients with OI who had been there because of the efforts of our members in the East. We spoke for a long time about his research and the important role the foundation was playing in it. Because of our letter-writing campaign, both of us felt optimistic that his grant would be renewed, and that someday, the pain Mike and the other children were experiencing would be alleviated.

A day or so after our accidental meeting at Shriners, Dr. Solomons' mood shifted drastically. In a dejected note, he wrote, "It was quite a shock to receive the enclosed letter, especially as previous communications from the NIH were optimistic." With his note was a copy of a letter from the National Institute of Arthritis and Metabolic Diseases informing him that his grant, though recommended for approval, was denied because of the unavailability of funds. He closed his letter with "I hope something can be done."

But what? What more could *we* do? Hadn't we already spent countless hours writing letters, making phone calls, holding meetings at our own expense and that of our families?

Disenchantment and biting recriminations from disappointed families followed news of the grant denial. "We were too slow, we weren't doing enough," some of the letters said. Others told us to leave them alone, quit promising them something we couldn't deliver. They had accepted OI as incurable until we had come along with our bright promises.

How cutting and hurtful the criticism was! Had I anticipated then all that was to follow, I surely would have thrown in the towel. But all these became inconsequential when on the heels of Dr. Solomons's note came word that my eldest brother had died suddenly of a heart attack at the age of fifty-four.

Irenee was my missionary brother who had spent over twenty years in Vietnam, then had come back to become rector of the Shrine of St. Anne de Beaupre in the Province of Quebec. It was he who had opened my eyes during my search for a miracle for Mike when he had told me, "Dear Gemma, it's supposed to hurt!"

After our return from his funeral at St. Anne's, I had to force myself to think about the foundation. My heart wasn't in it anymore. Some days, I just sat at my desk looking with dread at the piles of letters. I didn't want to read about other people's pains and problems, about their dashed hopes and dreams. I had enough sorrows of my own to cope with. Then one day, on top of the pile was a letter from Becky. This one I opened quickly, hoping to find in it the usual humor and encouragement.

The letter was only several lines, in which Becky had written, "Gemma, I have just sent Roy my resignation from the foundation. I know you will understand when I tell you that I arrived home from a few days vacation to find that my sister was tragically killed last night. I have her three orphaned children."

I read Becky's letter over and over again. To even think of continuing without her was more than I could bear. Tears sprang to my eyes for what Becky was going through, then it quickly turned to tears of self-pity for myself, for at that moment, I felt very much alone. I simply couldn't comprehend the loss of a promising research, an adored brother, and a much-needed friend all in one short week.

If it hadn't been for Renee and Roy and Mildred Burdette, I think that in the midst of our separate tragedies, Becky and I would surely have given up. But out of dedication to the cause, and because of a sincere affection for us, these three volunteered to augment their already heavy loads to give us a chance to cope with our grief. With their help, the work continued while we healed.

Late in August, a jubilant letter came from Roy and Mildred informing us that the Osteogenesis Imperfecta Foundation had been chartered on August 21, 1970. What a memorable milestone for all of us. Only a short while later, Dr. Solomons phoned to tell me that Shriners had renewed his grant and that there was a possibility that the NIH would give him a second opportunity to apply for government funding.

Then on a beautiful autumn day, I heard from Becky again. "Gemma, I think often of you and OIF and of the years gone by," she wrote. "The letters we have shared, the grief, the understanding, and the helping hands we share. Thank you, Gemma. How could I ever make it without you? How can we be such good friends just through letters?"

In that spirit, Becky was back. Her words made my heart lift, my spirits soar. Out loud, I said, "Thank *you*, Becky, Renee, Midge, Barbara, and all of you out there who believe in me. I could never have made it through these difficult times without all of you." Then to myself, I marveled, *Can it be true? Have all these wonderful things happened because of my story in Redbook?*

Chapter Twenty

The seventies were the best of times, the worst of times. The OI Foundation was flourishing under the direction of C. C. "Buck" McNeely, Jr., who had contacted us with an offer to help at the very moment when he had been needed the most. A savy corporate executive from North Carolina, Buck and his wife, Barbara, were the parents of a son Pat who had OI and was close to Mike's age. Our mutual concerns provided an immediate rapport that developed into a mentor-apprentice relationship that soon grew into a lasting friendship.

Buck had a wide range of experience on nonprofit boards, as well as the business know-how needed to operate a national organization. More importantly, he understood the value of the contributions our small mothers' group had made and encouraged us to continue using a personal approach by tempering the business aspects with compassion. So when Roy decided, after less than a year as president, to remain on the board but to volunteer his time in other capacities, there was no doubt in anyone's mind that Buck McNeely would be the perfect replacement.

With Buck's encouragement and guidance, I enlisted the help of Drs. Sofield and Millar and developed the first (to our knowledge) educational brochure about osteogenesis imperfecta. The day I held the finished pamphlet in my hands was a personal celebration for me. I couldn't help but think back to the day of Mike's birth when, unable to answer my questions, Dr. Burnes had surreptitiously placed a medical textbook with a few lines about OI on my bedside table. It had taken me a long time to find some of the answers, but here they were in my hands. Now other parents wouldn't have to take the long journey I'd taken in search of them.

Drs. Millar and Solomons were honored with a coveted scientific award, the Kappa Delta Award, for their joint paper "Osteogenesis imperfecta, New Perspectives in Diagnosis and Treatment." OI clinics were being established at major medical centers, and OIF's newly appointed Medical Advisory Board, headed by the distinguished Dr. Sofield, recommended funding the foundation's first research grant.

Sey Chassler, editor in chief of *Redbook*, published a progress report he'd asked me to write to let readers know what had happened as a result of "Epilogue to a Dream." This article, like the previous two, initiated another flood of letters and phone calls.

Because the mailing list for *Breakthrough* was growing too big, too fast for Becky and I to handle, Buck and his secretary at Burlington Industries took it over and computerized it by zip code for bulk mailing. I hired a printer in my hometown, and family and friends helped to package it for mailing. As a result, *Breakthrough* was developing into a professional-looking, well-respected newsletter with worldwide distribution.

Encouraged by OIF's success, a mother in Scotland told her story to newspapers and astonishingly got the same kind of response I'd received from my magazine pieces. With the help of Dr. Colin Paterson, Margaret Grant founded the Brittle Bone Society. From France came reports about research from J. P. Richard, an American father of an OI daughter working abroad. Wanting to become part of OIF, Canadians joined in with us, and parents from other countries began requesting guidelines for establishing their own OI organizations. By the end of the second year, OIF was reaching more people than had ever been imagined.

It was an almost euphoric time. I say almost because beneath the surface, there were continuous discontented rumblings from some of our own fledgling chapters who were threatening to break away and found their own organizations. It seemed that no matter what we did, it was never enough. It bothered me to think that the voluntary forty-hour weeks that some of us were putting in were not being appreciated. Buck assured me that all organizations experienced similar growing pains and that we should continue to strive to meet OIF goals without expecting to please everyone all the time.

Another piece of reality that dulled my exhilaration was my worry over Mike's restless desire to have the kind of life being enjoyed by his peers.

From Becky, Midge, and Renee, and many of the other parents who wrote regularly, I heard success stories. Most of their children were attending private or public schools, accompanied by their mothers or by special aides hired by and paid for by their school districts. Meanwhile, Mike's direct telephone hookup with school had become nearly obsolete.

A complicated diagram on the blackboard, a picture, a science experiment—none could be seen over a telephone wire. On rare occasions, some of the teachers came to our home to share a visual presentation with him, but it just wasn't enough. His schoolwork was going downhill fast, yet he was still getting good grades from his teachers. He didn't care or wonder anymore whether they were doing it because they felt sorry for him. Instead, he thought it kind of cool that he could get by so easily. More often than not, I'd catch him snoozing during class; he was so bored with the muffled sounds coming over the wire that were being presented to him as schooling.

Appalled, dismayed, and literally floored was what I was when one afternoon, while straightening up his room, I discovered a dog-eared *Playboy* magazine tucked inside one of his large notebooks. When I showed Dick my find the instant he came through the door, he laughed. "Calm down, honey. Mike's a teenage boy, and teenage boys are interested in stuff like that."

"Where could he have gotten it?" I lamented. "Do you suppose he has others stashed away?"

Dick took the magazine from me, flipped through the pages, and whistled softly. "Our little boy is definitely growing up. I guess I'd better have a talk with him."

OI teens and young adults had been writing to me about their concerns about sex and marriage, but I hadn't given much thought to the possibility that Mike might also be thinking about those things. The reason may have been that he was still child-sized, three feet tall, while his neighborhood friends had grown tall, were driving cars, and were dating. None of these things were happening for Mike, whose social life had dwindled so much that it now consisted mainly of hanging out with the younger kids who lived on our street.

After the startling *Playboy* incident, I decided to help Mike improve his social life by inviting a man who had OI and lived in a nearby town to come over to spend some time with him. In his late twenties or early thirties, the man had graduated from college, had an accounting business, and had boasted to me that he drove a car and had a girlfriend. Physically, he was no bigger than Mike. He'd be a good example, I thought, of what life with OI could be like. When I told Mike about the planned visit, he didn't appear interested but agreed to do it. However, when the day arrived, he mysteriously disappeared and was nowhere to be found. I suspected that he'd begged, even paid, his brother or one of the neighborhood kids to push his chair somewhere and hide him. When he reappeared almost immediately after our visitor had gone, he pretended having forgotten about the visit.

"You might have learned something from him about college, jobs, even women," I teased.

His eyes lit up momentarily; then he shrugged. "I don't want to be like him. I want . . ."

I waited to hear the rest, but he turned and wheeled away without finishing. He didn't have to continue. I knew what he wanted. He wanted to be like his able-bodied friends, his sisters, his brother, and everyone else.

I don't know how he would have survived those lonely teen years if he hadn't had his brother and sisters. Though our other children were involved in many extra curricular activities, they always managed to make Mike an important part of their everyday lives. Cathy attended the same high school as Mike did on his telephone hookup, so she carried his books and assignments back and forth and sometimes helped him with his homework. Having been there ahead of him, she was able to describe what his teachers looked like and what their expectations or peculiarities were. With Cindy, he shared an interest in rock music and the flower child movement that was going on at the time. A dreamy, envious look always crossed his face whenever they talked about rock concerts crowded with free-spirited hippies. Watching him, I told myself that he would have been there too, would have been one of them, had he been able.

His brother, Dick, had a lot of friends and was very involved in sports, yet it was Mike that he most often chose to be with. His close relationship with Dick made Mike feel wanted and needed. He was the senior member of the neighborhood gang now, and he relished teaching his younger brother and his friends the finer points of baseball . . . and other enterprises.

He was always scheming, trying to think of new and innovative things to do to while away the boredom. Long before the pet rock craze invaded the nation, I got a phone call one day from a neighbor. "Are you aware that some of the neighborhood kids are going door-to-door selling rocks?" she asked.

Laughing, I replied. "No, they haven't been here yet."

"They probably won't come to your house," she said. "They told me Mike put them up to it."

Outdoors, I found Mike sitting in his wheelchair, his dejected-looking group of young salesmen clustered around him, holding brown paper sacks filled with rocks.

Using my firm Mom voice and trying to keep a straight face, I said, "I hear you guys are selling rocks around the neighborhood."

Mike grinned. "Yes, well, we only sold one."

Wondering what kind soul had bought a rock, I told him. "I guess it was a bad idea, huh? Why don't you try a Kool-Aid stand instead?"

The younger boys cheered as Mike rolled his eyes in disgust to indicate that he was getting too old for that kid stuff. But quickly relenting, he said, "Well, okay, I'll help you guys, but only if Mom makes the Kool-Aid, and I get to collect the money." Like always, he would be making out on a deal without lifting a finger. And like his teachers, I let him get away with it because I felt bad about his inability to do the things his older friends were doing.

Years later, when pet rocks became the national craze, Mike loved to remind me that he'd been way ahead of the merchandisers with the idea of selling rocks and that he'd probably be a millionaire if I hadn't made him trade his great idea for a measly Kool-Aid stand.

Even though a lot of things in Mike's life were changing, his love of baseball remained constant. When his dad became involved coaching Dick's Little League team, Mike tagged along as his unofficial assistant. After each game, the three of them would rehash the game inning by inning and give young Dick pointers to improve his game. Early the next morning, the boys could be found on the backyard ball diamond trying out their strategies.

When they weren't practicing or playing ball, Mike and Dick were talking it, watching it on TV, swapping baseball cards, assessing the major leaguers, and recording batting averages and other statistics. Using a regular deck of playing cards, they devised a game around baseball that they played constantly. They were mini experts in every sport, but more so in baseball and football, and they relished predicting the outcome of major sporting events like the Indianapolis 500, the baseball All-Star

Game, the World Series, and the Super Bowl. These were events never to be missed at our house.

However, they nearly did miss one when we were on a motor trip to Canada on the very day that the all-star baseball game was being played. Fearful they would miss it, the boys had pestered their dad all day about stopping at a motel early enough to watch it on TV. So we had stopped early, had eaten quickly, showered, and had everyone in their pajamas ready to watch when we discovered that the only channel we could get was not broadcasting the game!

Undeterred, the boys asked their dad if they could listen to it on the car radio. But alas! This time the surrounding mountains interfered with the reception. Of course, that wouldn't do. So they talked their father into driving around until they found a hilltop where the game could be clearly heard. And there they sat for two hours, on a hilltop somewhere in the Province of Quebec, happily listening to the all-star game.

To fill the gaps that Mike's unusual mode of schooling left unsatisfied and to compensate the lack in his social life, we tried to encourage his passion and broaden his knowledge of sports by taking trips with the children to the National Baseball Hall of Fame in Cooperstown, New York, and the Pro Football Hall of Fame in Canton, Ohio. Occasionally, we took them to see Cincinnati Reds and Chicago Cubs baseball. Needless to say, those games were relived over and over again for weeks.

Camping and fishing were other activities that we all enjoyed, so we camped a lot. Though he seldom could go in the water because of cumbersome casts, Mike frequently went fishing for bluegills in our little green fishing boat with his dad and brother. In the evenings around the campfire, he was in his element, discussing not only sports, but world affairs, politics, and religion. He knew a lot about so many things and had strong opinions about those he cared about. Some of the radical statements he made about God and religion, I suspect, he made to shock us or to goad us into debates—another favorite pastime of his.

I often wondered how he knew so much about everything; he was so isolated. He read some and watched a lot of TV but, otherwise, had little exposure to the outside world other than through his less-than-adequate schooling and his interactions with us.

The way his brother and sisters so readily adjusted their own lives to bring some sort of normalcy to his reassured us that we must be doing something right. Like searching for the hilltop in Canada, they never stopped striving to make the things they took for granted possible for him.

One weekend, as we were preparing to leave our favorite campground, a woman who was staying at a neighboring campsite came over to talk to me. "At the start of the weekend, I watched your son in his wheelchair, and I was really impressed by the way he joined in with the other children instead of sitting on the sidelines," she said.

I smiled. She sounded so much like everyone else who had a chance to observe fun-loving Mike.

Taking a deep breath, she continued. "I hope you won't take this the wrong way, but now that the weekend is over, my admiration has shifted to the other children in the family."

"Oh?" I said, pleasantly surprised to hear that our other children had finally been noticed.

"I don't know how many times your younger son helped his brother bait his fish hook, not to mention all the times he pushed his wheelchair around the baseball field! And the girls—they must have walked to the camp store a dozen times to buy him something or other. And they did it so patiently, so lovingly. I just had to tell you what a good feeling it gave me to watch them."

No matter how hard they tried, there were some things our other children weren't able to change. They especially dreaded it when Mike had to be admitted to Shriners Hospital, over two hundred miles away, for months at a time. They missed him and hated not being allowed to enter the hospital to visit him. Cindy, who had been Mike's rescuer from the time she could walk, once told me, "I remember how we stood by the big fence that surrounded the hospital courtyard, our eyes glued to the door, watching and waiting to see if Mike would be allowed to come out. And when finally he did come out, we would jump up and down with joy and call his name. We tried to cram in as many smiles and as much laughter as we could during those brief visits. But what stands out most in my mind, when I remember, was the pain I felt because I couldn't rescue him and bring him home."

The hospital, like school, had serious barriers to overcome. Thanks to Dr. Millar and the OI clinic nurse, my friend Frances Dubowski, the hospital was working to remove them. The school barriers we would have to continue tackling on our own.

While discussing Mike's fall schedule with the principal the spring he finished his sophomore year, it became abundantly clear that there were few opportunities of learning left open to him in the coming year. Most of the subjects required and/or available were subjects that concentrated mainly of laboratory work, languages, and cooperative work-study programs like the one Cathy had taken her last two years of high school. Since the school was a three-story structure without elevators, we were told that the only subject that Mike hadn't already taken that was physically accessible to him was drafting.

Luckily, Mike had always enjoyed drawing and design and wanted to try drafting. With some persuasion, the principal finally agreed to enroll him in this class for one forty-three-minute period a day, but only if we took the responsibility of transporting him to and from school. The remainder of his classes would have to be over the intercom as usual.

Though he hadn't grown much in height, Mike had steadily gained weight and was becoming too heavy for me to lift as often as would be necessary to transport him back and forth to school. His admittance meant that we had to devise a means of letting him get in and out of the car by himself with a minimum of help. Using a helpful hint on how to bridge the gap between wheelchair and car seat sent to OIF by another parent, Dick took a four-foot board, sanded it, and varnished it well so Mike could easily slide out of his wheelchair and onto the car seat. With his lightweight wheelchair folded, both the board and chair could then be lifted into the car trunk without too much strain.

Mike appeared nervous his first day of school. For the first time in his life, he would be going into a normal school situation. Many of the classmates he had taken intercom classes with would be seeing him for the first time, and he worried about how they would react to his short stature and useless legs. He needn't have worried. Most of the young people were wonderful and treated him the same as everyone else.

Relieved, Mike used all the energy he could muster during the forty-three minutes he was at school trying to catch up on everything he'd missed, especially the socializing. He also worked harder than usual and tried to concentrate more effort on the subject that is sometimes just a schedule filler for some but that for him might mean a future opportunity to become employed. He had to learn to work in a group situation, to keep pace with his peers in the so-called normal world. And he desperately wanted and needed to cultivate friendships.

At home, he spent hours at the drafting board that had been loaned to him by a local corporation. On it, he drew a variety of plans for his future home. They were crude designs, but they encompassed all his hopes and dreams.

"Are there going to be any children in that dream house?" I once asked.

Gruffly, he replied, "I'd better find a wife first. Don't you think?"

"Don't worry. You'll find one," I told him reassuringly. Then I repeated for him the stories I'd told him time and time again about some of the married individuals I was getting to know and admire—persons with OI like Nelda Roehm and her husband, Jack. And Pete Moore, billed as the smallest man in the world, yet happily married and the father of two children.

Sometimes he'd respond with a joke about the remoteness of the possibilities I painted for him, but there were times when I saw in his eyes the dim hope that maybe, just maybe, it could happen to him too.

Chapter Twenty-One

I was about to go out the door one evening on my way to give a talk to a group of church women when Dick called me to the phone. "It's one of your critics," he whispered as he handed me the phone.

"You should have told him I wasn't here!" I hissed.

He shrugged helplessly. "He said it was important. I thought you might want to hear what he has to say."

"It's okay. I'll take it," I said, giving my ever-patient husband a forgiving smile.

It was a long, depressing phone call during which my critic advised me for the hundredth time to start paying attention to the demands of our discontented members; otherwise, they would surely splinter from OIF and compete with it for the research dollars we were trying to raise.

By the time the phone call ended, I was in absolutely no mood to bare my heart and soul to a bunch of strangers, much less speak positively about everything that OIF was accomplishing. If perchance my caller was right and we were wrong, soon there wouldn't be an OIF to brag about!

It was way past the time I'd been scheduled to speak. Hurriedly, I drove through darkened streets toward the home of the young woman where I was to deliver my speech. I was a veteran speechmaker by then, a celebrity of sorts who was in much demand. I hadn't had an episode of stage fright since the one in the OI clinic room at Shriners the day we had founded OIF. So why was my stomach churning? Why was I feeling so nauseous and light-headed? This sick, uncomfortable feeling should have been reason enough to turn around and go home. But on the seat beside me were my wonderful handouts—OIF brochures and copies of *Breakthrough*—the public awareness tools that I had so proudly developed and were still so needed, even here in our town where everyone knew our family's story.

The women waiting for me in the brightly lighted living room were friendly and receptive. Relaxing, I chatted with them as I passed out my handouts. I had barely started speaking when suddenly the room began to spin violently. Then came a feeling of being caught up in a cyclone that offered no escape. Desperately, I tried to keep talking as I had done the other time in Chicago, tried to find something to hold on to steady myself. But Midge, Becky, and Renee weren't there to support me, and the spinning continued until I began to perspire heavily and became so nauseous. I had to ask directions to the bathroom where I repeatedly vomited as some of the concerned mothers watched from the doorway.

Sounding petrified, one of them said, "She must be having a heart attack. We should call an ambulance!"

"I'm not having a heart attack," I managed to say. "Please, don't call an ambulance. Call my husband. He'll come to take me home."

Appearing worried, they nevertheless did as I asked, and in no time at all, Dick was there with Cathy and Cindy. Quickly, they gathered up my belongings. Dick helped me into his car, and Cathy got into the car I had driven to take it home.

Sounding scared, but in command, Dick said, "They think you might have had a heart attack. I'm taking you to the hospital."

"I'm *not* having a heart attack," I insisted as the world continued to whirl around me. "I'm so embarrassed, I just want to go home."

"Please, Mom, let Dad take you to the hospital," Cindy pleaded from the backseat.

"No, not the hospital," I begged.

Reluctantly, they gave in to my wishes. "Okay, we'll take you home, but I'm calling the doctor as soon as we get there," Dick said.

Agreeing, I limply surrendered to the unrelenting spinning.

After examining me, our doctor diagnosed an inner ear infection as the cause of my dizziness and gave me an injection and some medication to tame it. He said it would probably be a few days before I would feel steady again and advised bed rest.

I doubted the inner ear infection diagnosis. If it was correct, why had I only been plagued on the two occasions when a speech had followed a demoralizing bout of criticism? Could it be that these personal attacks were causing my fragile inner self to react with so much turbulence it had to outwardly manifest itself? I wondered, but accepted the doctor's simpler explanation and did as he ordered.

The next morning, Dick carried me to the living room couch and gently ordered me not to do anything resembling work while he and the children were gone. Mike would be at home, and he assured his father that he would keep a close eye on me. I didn't tell them, but I couldn't have done anything anyway. Just remembering how I had humiliated myself the night before was enough to make me dizzy and nauseous all over again.

Sometime around midmorning, I woke up from a short nap to find Mike stationed next to the couch in his wheelchair.

"You don't have to guard me this close. I'm not going anywhere," I joked feebly.

He didn't laugh, didn't even smile. I could tell by the look on his face that he'd been contemplating something serious, but I felt too tired for one of our lively debates, so I turned away and closed my eyes.

Realizing my weariness, he spoke softly, "Why do you do it, Mom? Why do you put yourself through this torture, taking all that bullshit from those people who phone and criticize everything you're trying to do?"

I sighed. "Sometimes I ask myself the same thing."

"If you're doing it for me, then don't," he ventured. "I'm sick of having all that OI stuff around, of being reminded of it constantly. Can't we forget about it for a while? Live our own lives like everyone else?"

Had I heard him right? "Forget about OI?" I countered back. "How can we forget it? You have to live with it . . . *we* have to live with it day in and day out. And to answer your first question, I guess I do what I do with the hope that it will make things easier and better for you . . . and us, and all those other children and parents. Maybe I don't want to stop, can't stop . . ." I wailed as I eased my spinning head back onto a pillow.

"Then it's all yours. You can have it!" he announced vehemently. His voice cracking a little, he added, "I just don't want you getting sick over this on account of me, that's all." And as he often did after a serious discussion, he wheeled away to his room to reflect on what he had said.

When he came back later to check on me, he appeared contrite. "Don't think I don't care about everything you've done," he said. "It's just that . . ."

"I promise not to involve you anymore, if you don't want me to," I offered. "And I won't write about you. And I'm definitely not making anymore speeches. But I can't and won't stop everything else I'm doing."

"Mom, I shouldn't have said what I did. It wasn't fair."

"It's okay. I understand," I said, and I did understand to a certain extent.

From the first day of his forty-three-minutes-a-day stint at school, I had seen him trying to pull away from us, to break free of all the restrictions that had been imposed on him since birth because of osteogenesis imperfecta. He wanted to be like his new friends, to do what they were doing, and go wherever they were going.

One day, when driving down one of our busiest streets, I saw his friend Russell zigzagging through traffic on his bike. Holding on to the back of the bike, his hair blowing in the breeze, was our fragile Mike in his wheelchair. Trembling, I pulled my car to the curb until I was calm enough to drive again. Later, when I mentioned the incident to Nelda Roehm, a friend who has OI, her response was "Let him be. He's reaching for his independence."

"But he could have been killed," I cried.

Matter-of-factly, she replied, "Then he would have died a free person."

For several months, I'd been confiding in Nelda by phone about the new challenges we were encountering with Mike. Nelda had acquired a wealth of information about OI, but most importantly, she seemed to have an inborn source of knowledge about the way the minds of OI teens and young adults worked. Having fought fiercely for her own independence from overprotective parents, and being married with a life of her own, she could zero in on a problem and help me solve it or accept it.

Like Buck McNeely, Nelda had come into my life and on the OIF scene at a time when she was most needed. Becky's position as secretary had been filled for a short while by Carol Gortat of Illinois, then for several terms by Mildred Burdette. A prolific letter writer who knew other OI adults, Nelda was the undisputed choice when Mildred chose to resign.

When Becky began drifting away to become more involved in Doug's schooling and other family matters, and when Midge decided to leave the board to become more active in chapter and support group activities in Michigan, I gravitated toward Nelda, even though Renee and I were still close coworkers and good friends.

By then, I was second vice president as well as *Breakthrough* editor. Being secretary, Nelda wrote or phoned often with stories about families who were contacting OIF and about their particular medical needs or coping problems. Hours were spent trying to figure out where to refer them for medical attention, what to do about cases of suspected child abuse that we knew to be OI, or how to handle the emotional topic of child deaths and other sensitive issues in *Breakthrough*.

Both Nelda and I felt that persons with OI should be honestly depicted as real people who happened to have "brittle bones," and not as saints or heroic figures who were always sweet, courageous, and perfect as they were so often portrayed by the media.

Saddened by the death of Bob and Norma Lutzinger's little daughter, Jennifer, we felt the need to mention in *Breakthrough* the children who had died so we could grieve openly with their parents. This was done within the context of a memorial column developed and sensitively written by Doris Krebs, a mother who had lost an OI baby boy.

We wanted teens and young adults to feel comfortable reading about and discussing concerns and questions about dating and marriage— subjects most parents avoided with their OI teens. Talking about some of the things Mike and some of the other teens were going through made us realize how much they would benefit if they could meet and talk openly about these hushed-up subjects with adults who had survived the unique pains of growing up with OI. Thus, the idea of a national conference for teens and young adults with OI was born.

Because some members of the board opposed exploring feelings in print, we published medical articles instead. At my request, Dr. Millar wrote "An Explanation of Rodding Surgery," and Frances Dubowski, RN, researched and wrote a pamphlet on "The Care of an OI Baby and Child." These two pieces of literature were and continue to be among those most often requested by parents and professionals.

To my delight, I was becoming more knowledgeable about the medical aspects of OI and was reading all the research papers I could get my hands on. Aware of this, Nelda kept me supplied with transcripts of every medical speech made and every medical research paper published. I found them intriguing and fairly easy to understand. Dr. Solomon's magnesium oxide treatment, I discovered, hadn't been the only one tried. In fact, between 1911 and 1940, articles about vitamin D had predominated. Then between 1930 and 1968, androgens and estrogens had been tried. Also in the late sixties, the effects of fluoride had been studied. And since 1972, not only magnesium oxide, but also calcitonin, a hormone with direct effect on bone, was being tried.

The renewed interest in OI research in clinical settings and in laboratories around the world prompted Dr. Millar to invite thirty OI researchers to Shriners Hospital for what was believed to be the first such meeting in the history of the study of OI—an international symposium to evaluate research projects and studies and the medications and treatments being used. I felt quite privileged to be among those invited and happier still that I'd done my homework and was able to understand most of the topics presented. I could hardly wait to get back home so I could put everything I'd heard to good use.

Gradually, I was also learning to concentrate more on the larger OI picture by giving more attention to research and the experiences of others rather than those of the Geisman family. In the Feelings column that was eventually approved, I explored coping topics without using our experiences and adventures with Mike as focal points.

I was doing my best to honor my promise to Mike to let him live his own life without compromising my involvement in the OIF work I'd come to love so much.

Chapter Twenty-Two

Letting Mike live his own life was easier said than done. The problem being that we couldn't come to terms about how he should live it.

Cathy had married a few months after her high school graduation and was expecting a baby. Though Cindy was only seventeen, she couldn't wait to be off to college and was trying to cram high school into three years instead of the usual four.

Not about to be left behind, Mike constantly reminded us that he too would be leaving soon. "I'll be moving out after graduation. I'll be eighteen then, so you won't be able to stop me," he'd challenge, then watch for a reaction.

Not fully realizing how determined he was, we humored him by telling him that we did agree that moving out on his own was indeed a great idea!

Not convinced that we meant it, he'd argue back, "You don't really think I can do it, do you?"

We didn't think he *could* or *would* do it, but knowing that he would be even more determined to leave if he knew we doubted his ability to become independent, we tried to answer "Of course, we think you can!" with some conviction.

Alone in bed at night was another matter. Night after night, Dick and I agonized over Mike's great need for independence and our even greater fear of letting him go. So obsessed were we with this ongoing discussion that nothing else seemed to matter. That is, until Cathy, whose husband was stationed away with the army, asked if she could stay with us for the remainder of her pregnancy. Though this was a happy diversion, for the most part, the presence of osteogenesis imperfecta in our lives did cause us some concerns about the expected baby.

Mike too was worried. One day, when he and I were alone, he asked, "Mom, could Cathy's baby have OI like me?"

"It's possible, but not likely," I responded as lightly as I could.

Sucking in his breath, he said, "God, I hope not." Then he wheeled himself to his room to face the likelihood alone.

Toward the end of her pregnancy, Cathy became subdued and thoughtful. She seemed to be struggling with some inner fear, and I sensed that she too was worried that her baby might be born with OI.

Long before their marriage, I had spoken to Cathy and her husband-to-be, Charlie, about getting genetic counseling, but they hadn't. Now all the possibilities and percentages loomed, and it was difficult not to think about them.

Her voice trembling, Cathy finally put her fears into words. "Mom, what am I going to do if our baby is born with OI?"

My breath caught. I wanted to say, "Don't worry. It won't happen." Instead, I instructed her to remind our new family doctor, who was to deliver her baby, about Mike's condition so that he would be alerted to immediately check the baby at birth for symptoms of the disorder. I also explained gently that a great deal more was now known about OI and that better care facilities were available. In the event that the improbable did happen, I assured her that I would use all the resources at my disposal to get the best care for her child.

We never discussed OI again during the remainder of her pregnancy even though it was uppermost in our minds as the day of delivery neared. Then at last, at dawn on the first day of spring, a perfect baby girl they named Jennifer was born.

We cried, all of us, when we saw her red and wrinkly, naked and screaming on the nursery scales. She was the most beautiful sight in the world—our granddaughter.

We enjoyed Jennifer for a few short months until she and her mother flew off to Germany to be with her daddy. Soon after they'd gone, Mike again began rumbling about leaving as soon as he graduated.

The evening he finally did graduate, dressed in a gray cap and gown that had to be cut in half to fit him, should have been one of the happiest moments of his life. All the ingredients for a perfect occasion were in place. A warm, pleasant June evening, a standing ovation as Dick pushed his chair to the podium for him to receive his diploma, a party with lots of gifts and tributes afterward—all this should have been more than enough to mark this important milestone. And that evening, Mike did appear to be enjoying it all. However, several days later, while I was helping him sort out the congratulatory cards and presents, he asked, "Why do you think they gave me a standing ovation? Was it because they felt sorry for me? I didn't do anything to deserve it, yet some of the kids who really worked hard barely got any applause at all."

I understood what he was saying because the standing ovation had reminded me somewhat of the overly sympathetic teachers who had given him grades he hadn't earned because they had felt sorry for him. But not wanting to spoil the memory of his graduation, I pushed those thoughts aside and told him, "I don't think the standing ovation was about grades. I think it was the audience's way of telling you that they admired you for sticking it out against all odds."

"You think so?" he asked, but didn't appear convinced.

"Yes," I responded firmly.

"Well, whatever the reason, I didn't like being singled out like that. Accepting all that applause with a smile made me feel like a hypocrite and a fraud!"

Only a few weeks later, Mike would again experience the indignation of being singled out for what he believed to be the wrong reasons.

The summer had started off on a very dull note. Cathy and Jennifer were gone. Cindy was taking summer classes and working. Young Dick was active in PONY League Baseball and not around much anymore to play sandlot ball with Mike and the neighborhood kids. A few friends still came around on occasion, but most were busy with jobs and girlfriends. When several of his buddies asked if he'd be interested in coaching a Little League team with them, Mike perked up considerably. We all knew that he was practically an expert when it came to baseball and that he loved teaching the little kids how to play, so we wholeheartedly encouraged him to do it.

I'll never forget the happy look on his face the day he went to the tryouts with his friends, his Chicago Cubs hat planted firmly on his head, his notepad held tightly under his arm.

After they had played a few games, Mike became the team strategist, spending hours after every game, figuring out what had worked and what hadn't, working on the lineup, phoning the kids to remind them of practices and game times and other related information. Often, I'd overhear him counseling a boy on the other end of the line, encouraging him or helping him to understand the game. When he thought some of the other coaches (mostly all fathers of boys who were playing) were breaking league rules, he'd call the head of the league to protest, an activity that probably led to what happened next.

Several of the fathers who coached were especially loud and obnoxious and often engaged in shouting matches with some of the other coaches or umpires. During one particular game, Mike made the deadly mistake of engaging in one of those shouting matches with them, using the same choice words they were using. Not long after the incident, he was told by a league official that he could no longer coach. When he asked whether the other coaches were also being suspended, he was told that they were not and that the shouting match was not the reason he was being relieved of his team. The real reason, he was told, was that some of the parents found it inappropriate to have a handicapped kid, who was smaller than their sons and had never played organized baseball, doing the coaching. Devastated, Mike admitted that he'd been wrong to shout and argue in front of the players and begged to be given another chance to prove that he could coach. But he was denied the chance. When Dick protested to league officials, they told him they would allow Mike to coach again only if he, Dick, became the team's head coach. By then, Dick had obtained his license to umpire and had a very busy schedule that left him no time for coaching, so he had to decline the offer. Mike said he didn't care for that arrangement anyway since they weren't making the offer because of his coaching ability, but simply to pacify his dad, who had given years of service to the league. "I'm not coaching anymore because I don't look the part and that's that," he said bitterly.

I was upset at Mike for spoiling his chance to coach by engaging in unsportsmanlike conduct, but I was equally disturbed about the fact that the other coaches had not been reprimanded in any way. However, it was the other reasons given for his dismissal that hurt the most. Had he been given another chance, I knew that Mike could have been one of the best coaches the league had ever had even though he was physically smaller than the boys he coached and had to maneuver around the ball field in a wheelchair.

Some of the boys on Mike's team were also unhappy with the loss of their coach, and they took to coming over to our house to hang out and talk baseball with him. Though he appreciated their loyalty, his heart wasn't in it anymore. Now more than ever, all he could think about was getting away from the dictates, restrictions, and prejudices that controlled his life.

Because he was feeling at loose ends, he agreed with his rehab counselor that now was a good time for him to go to a job training center in Fort Wayne, Indiana, for the job skills evaluation he had turned down a few weeks earlier.

When we visited him there, he did nothing but complain that the place was depressing and that the staff didn't understand anything about him. They were insistent, he said, that he should train to do the same kind of boring, menial work that their mentally disabled clients were doing or else use his mathematical skills to study accounting. They urged him to get realistic and said that his hope of getting into radio broadcasting was a pipe dream, that rehab would never approve. Given these choices, he naturally opted for accounting and was enrolled to begin fall classes at a university branch in Lima, Ohio.

Several days after returning from Fort Wayne, he casually mentioned one afternoon that he was going for a walk to think things over. Going for a walk usually meant wheeling his wheelchair on the sidewalk for several blocks, then back. When he had been gone for several hours, I went looking for him, but he was nowhere in sight. Fearing that he'd gone too far and couldn't get back or, even worse, that he'd tipped his chair off a curb and was lying hurt somewhere, I got in the car and began driving around looking for him. Unable to find him, I returned home and began phoning some of his friends. Those I was able to reach hadn't seen him or wouldn't tell me if they had. Cindy and Dick hadn't seen him either. By the time his father got home, I was imagining all sorts of terrible accidents. Though he was worried too, Dick tried to reassure me. "Some of his friends must have picked him up, and he's probably out joyriding, having a high old time while you're worrying yourself sick. He'll turn up."

He was right. Mike finally did turn up, looking grimy and tired three days later! I exploded after the friend, who had dropped him off, had gone. "Where have you been?" I cried. "We called everyone, searched everywhere for you! You could have let us know you were still alive!" I began to sob. "I imagined you dead somewhere in a ditch!"

Looking contrite, he murmured, "I guess I botched this up too. I'm sorry, Mom, but I just had to get away to think things through."

"So you said," I replied. "But you could have told us you wanted to go away. We could have helped . . ."

"I'm tired of you and Dad helping me with everything. I wanted to do this on my own."

Still angry, I probed, "Where were you?"

"Where I was doesn't matter. All that should matter is that I'm back."

I softened. "Mike, next time . . . if there's a next time, at least call us and let us know you're okay. I don't think we could take another three days of not knowing."

The rest of the family reacted much the same as I had when they came home and found that he had returned. They told him how angry they were at him for disappearing without a word, but they also made sure that he knew they were relieved and happy to have him back unharmed. But no matter how much we quizzed him about where he'd been, he wouldn't say. Weeks later, one of his friends confessed to me that he'd let Mike sleep in his car at night after they'd spent the daytime hours unsuccessfully searching for an apartment to rent with his graduation money.

Not long after his disappearing act, Mike took off again, this time in a car with one of his buddies. Later that day, he phoned to say that he'd been over to talk to his grandmother and that she had agreed that he could move in with her until he found his own place. If I didn't mind, he said, he'd be over later with several of his friends to pack his things.

Even though I knew that Mike's moving out was a desperate attempt to become independent, I felt deeply hurt that he had chosen to live with his grandmother rather than to stay with us, but I tried not to sound it. I suspected that Dick's mother had taken him in to spare us a repeat of the last ordeal. Another redeeming factor was that I knew that with her, he would be loved and cared for. "Come on over. I'll help you pack," I said gaily and hung up.

By the end of the summer, he was back home again. With no questions asked, we took him in and helped him find transportation back and forth to Lima for his first semester of college. He'd only been in college a matter of weeks when he triumphantly announced that a local bank had approved his application for a college loan and that he'd rented an apartment and was moving out on his own.

The apartment was in a nice neighborhood on the first floor below an elderly woman's apartment. We highly approved his choice of a quiet place to study, and being ever so grateful that he'd finally found what he had been looking for, we helped him to move in. It wasn't long, however, before our image of Mike studying in quiet solitude was completely shattered.

In the wee hours of a Sunday morning, only weeks after Mike had moved, the insistent ringing of the phone jolted us out of bed. On the phone, sounding very distraught, was the elderly tenant who lived above Mike's apartment. "Your boy is having a wild party downstairs. People have been coming in and out all night. I called down there and asked them to turn down the music and the noise so I could sleep, but whoever answered was very rude and hung up on me. You'd better do something, or I'm going to call the police!"

"I'll take care of it," Dick assured her. He hung up and quickly dialed Mike's number, but got no response. "Either it's so noisy in there that they can't hear the phone, or else they think it's the upstairs tenant, and they're not answering it. I guess I'll have to get dressed and go over there."

Even though I really didn't want to go, I asked, "Do you want me to go with you?"

"No, you stay here. I won't be long," he said.

When he returned a while later, he was very angry. "The music was blasting so loud, I could hear it a mile away! The apartment was in shambles, and some of his friends were either asleep or passed out. I don't know which!"

"And Mike? What about him?"

"Oh, he was having a great time, said he'd only invited a few friends, but that word of a party got around and that a lot of uninvited people showed up. When I ordered everyone out, he got very upset and told me to get out and mind my own business."

"Did you? Get out, I mean?"

"No, I stayed. Turned the music off and got everyone out." He paused, then sounding more hurt than angry, he said, "Mike really hates me now for interfering . . . and right now, I don't like him very much either."

Sighing, I replied, "This was his first real chance to be independent, and he blew it. Do you think he'll get kicked out of the apartment?"

"Probably," Dick responded glumly.

Wanting to smooth things over, I said, "He was only having a party the same as most guys do when they get their first apartment. Maybe it wasn't his fault it got out of hand."

"Maybe not. But you forget that most people don't think of him as an adult because of his size. To them, he's still a fragile little boy in a wheelchair, and they can't imagine him doing normal adult male things, and we're still the Mom and Dad responsible for what he does." Then sounding very tired, he said, "Let's try to get some sleep. We'll try to talk some sense into him tomorrow."

After Dick had fallen asleep, I remained sleepless until dawn wondering whether I was responsible for having created a public image of Mike that wasn't the flesh and blood person he really was. In the end, I decided that I had always tried to honestly portray Mike, and that the way others perceived him and other disabled individuals was not my doing, but that of generations before me.

Wide awake with nothing else to occupy me, I organized an article in my mind about the many things a parent could do to alter the misconceptions the public had about children with disabilities. Years would pass before I would finally write it and have it published in a well-respected parenting publication. In the meantime, Dick and I still had much to learn about parenting a disabled male adult bent on achieving his personal independence, no matter what the cost.

Chapter Twenty-Three

The OI Foundation, like Mike, was suffering growing pains that were becoming difficult to cope with. By now, two of our chapters on the East Coast had broken away from OIF to become autonomous, competing organizations. Others who admired their feistiness and "big-time" ideas were threatening to do the same. What bothered me most about the split was that with them had gone some of the members we had located and painstakingly cultivated. Several, who encouraged the divisiveness, were researchers whom we had enthusiastically supported. Others were members of OI families who had used up a great deal of our time and energy with their problems.

Had the maverick groups gone amicably, it would have been easier to understand. But they hadn't. Instead, they had written letters to board members that were meant to create doubts about the competence of those of us who were in charge. I was sometimes referred to as the little housewife or young mother from Ohio who meant well but didn't have the know-how required to be a member of the team working to establish a very complex national organization. OIF was labeled a "kitchen table" operation that needed to move out into the real world to compete with other nonprofits for hard-to-get research money.

Even after they had severed all ties with OIF, the dissidents continued to openly criticize the foundation policies and did all they could to sway the sentiments of those who remained loyal to OIF.

Often, during those troublesome times, I'd ask myself the same question Mike had once asked. *Why are you putting up with all that bullshit? You don't need or deserve any of this on top of everything else!*

Everything else included not only Mike's escapades but the realization that the cleaning business Dick and I had worked so hard to build was becoming a casualty of the recession that was critically affecting the Midwest. *Or was it my fault?* I wondered. *Had I been spending too much time trying to locate OI families instead of potential customers? Were the hours spent on OI-related phone calls causing us to lose incoming business calls?* My hardworking husband assured me that I had owned up to my responsibilities as his business partner, that the decline in business was due to the poor economy of the times and not to anything I had neglected to do. Still, I worried and felt guilty about it. So when we finally closed down the business and Dick went to work in a factory that manufactured steel buildings, I found work as a part-time bookkeeper for a small women's apparel shop. My intentions were to begin phasing OIF out of my life so I could eventually become employed full-time. Already, college expenses were making a dent in our tight budget, and soon, young Dick would also be off to college.

But my intentions of leaving OIF work behind didn't pan out. Instead, I was elected president and became even more involved. At the request of his colleagues on the executive board, Buck agreed to stay on in the second vice president position so we could avail ourselves of his expertise. Renee, who was first vice president, took charge of the growing number of state area coordinators, chapters, and support groups. Bob Krebs of Virginia replaced Roy as treasurer; Nelda hired a part-time secretary to help with the increasing volume of mail; and Janice Wadstrom, an OI woman from Connecticut, became the new *Breakthrough* editor. I couldn't have asked for a more caring, more dedicated team. Yet even with all the additional help, my own workload increased dramatically.

Working away from home for part of the day, I now spent many late-evening hours, after the rest of the family had gone to bed, catching up on OIF business by writing memos and letters and by making and receiving phone calls that came at all hours, like the one that jogged me out of bed one morning at 3:00 a.m.

As I picked up the phone, I heard a woman sobbing, "I can't do it anymore! I thought I could, but now I know I can't!"

Still groggy with sleep, I mumbled, "What can't you do anymore?"

"I can't take care of this baby one more day!" she cried. "My husband is always away at work, my friends have deserted me . . . I'm alone for hours with him, worrying and wondering whether he'll break the next time I pick him up to feed him or change his diaper. I'm so afraid he'll die, yet sometimes I think we'd all be better off if he did . . ."

Her ambivalence and confusion jolted me back to the days when, like her, I had felt alone and unable to cope one more day with the burden of responsibility that had been foisted on me. "I had the same feelings once," I whispered into the phone. "And I still hurt bad sometimes when I can't understand the things Mike and the rest of my family are going through. But now I have people helping me, supporting me."

"But I don't!" she wailed.

"Yes, you do," I replied firmly. "You have me and the resources of the OI Foundation at your disposal. Please, try to get some sleep. I'll call you back tomorrow and give you the names of doctors and parent contacts in your area. I'll send you literature . . . and anything else you may need."

There was a hopeful lilt in her voice when she asked, "You won't forget? You will call me tomorrow for sure?"

I assured her that I wouldn't forget and hung up. When I went back to bed, Dick stirred. "I hope that wasn't another call about Mike," he said with apprehension.

"No, it was an OIF call."

Raising up on an elbow, he grumbled, "In the middle of the night! Honey, this has got to stop! You have to cut these nighttime hours out!"

"I'll try," I promised, but in my heart, I knew that the probability that I would keep that pledge was slim since I couldn't bring myself to limit my work, especially my responses to such desperate cries for help. Besides, because of the time differences between continents, calls from Europe and Australia were coming in at odd hours, as were those from the Western states.

In Australia, Kerry Kenihan, a writer who wrote regularly for women's magazines, had given birth to Quentin, who was severely affected with OI. Kerry and her husband, Geoff, who was also a journalist, had agreed shortly after Quentin's birth to share their story with the readers of a popular Australian women's magazine. The response to their story had been similar to the responses from my *Redbook* pieces and to Margaret Grant's stories, and it had encouraged the Kenihans to establish the Australian OI Foundation.

As had happened with Margaret Grant of Scotland, the Kenihans and I soon became friends, and one of the first items of business I handled as OIF president was a request for financial aid from the Australian OI Foundation to help bring Dr. Solomons to Australia. Our Medical Advisory Board approved the grant, and Solomons was off to Australia. While there, he made sixteen presentations to scientists, clinicians, and allied health personnel in Melbourne, Sidney, Adelaide, and Canberra and began an attempt to integrate treatment and research there with similar activities as in the United States.

Subsequently, I planned an executive board meeting, the second since the organizational meeting, to discuss future goals. The first executive board meeting had been called by Buck at the McNeely's North Carolina seashore home and had been very energizing. This one, hosted by Don and Renee in their Alabama home, did not turn out to be the affirmative session we had planned. The damper was a visit from the determined parents of an OI child from Minnesota whom I had invited with the hope that they would take on leadership roles within OIF. Instead, nearly all their time with us was taken up with a long list of things they felt we were doing wrong, along with the steps they thought we should take to correct them. After hearing them out, we politely thanked them for coming, then proceeded to point out the many things *we* thought we were doing right. They went home feeling that we had let them down, and eventually, they joined one of the chapters that had split from OIF and formed a separate organization. We left Alabama more determined than ever not to let our critics destroy what had been accomplished and what was planned for the future of OIF. Our connections in Europe and Australia, our growing network of volunteers in America, and the research spreading around the world was proof enough for us that we were headed in the right direction. For me, these positives were also the remedies needed to counteract my growing disillusionment with Mike's antics.

To all outward appearances, I was handling things well. My correspondence with members was positive and upbeat. Other than Buck and Nelda, I told no one—not even Renee, Becky, and Midge—that Mike had dropped out of college and had been kicked out of a growing number of apartments because of his loud parties.

My friends' sons were doing so well. Donny Gardner was attending college, driving a car, and coaching baseball. Doug Keller was getting all sorts of scholastic awards and honors. And Mark Peck was already halfway through college and planning to attend law school. How could I confide to them what was happening with Mike?

Between apartments, Mike had moved back home on several occasions. During those times, he and I spent endless hours in prolonged discussions, hashing things out as he called it. Most of the time, he talked, and I listened. *If I paid strict attention*, I told myself, *maybe I'd be able to figure out what was wrong and find a way to fix it.*

He couldn't hack college, he said. He'd been caught snoozing during class; it was so boring. The professors spoke too fast during their lectures. His mind could absorb what they said, but his notetaking couldn't keep up. Why did he have to take accounting anyway when all he wanted was to be a disc jockey or radio sports announcer? He said he'd been talking to his rehab counselor about finding a job instead of going back to college, but so far, nothing had turned up, so he was making do with the small SSI check the government was sending him every month.

Once, at the end of another fruitless discussion, I asked, "Mike, have you tried praying for help?"

His face grew taunt. "Pray? Pray to who? The one who made me like this?" he sneered and spread out his short twisted arms for me to see. "No thanks. As far as I'm concerned, there is no God. And even if there is, I'll gladly do without his help!"

I had no comforting words for him. Lately, I too had been having doubts of my own about the power of prayer, yet I persisted with my prayerful questions. "God, I'm working so hard for other OI people, why can't you at least show me how to help Mike?"

When there came no response or evidence that God had heard me, I tried not to despair openly. Instead, I kept feeding Mike hope by telling him that if he seriously applied himself, someday he would have all that he desired—an independent life, a job or career, and a home and family.

Believing that what I told him could come true, he picked himself up many times to try again. He thought he was finally on his way when his rehab counselor found him a late-afternoon/early-evening bookkeeping job at the local YWCA.

He was living with us at the time, and since I promised to transport him to his job every day, he decided to stay put. It took some coaxing, but he agreed to cut the hair that he'd let grow to shoulder length and to trim the beard he had grown so people wouldn't mistake him for a child. He agreed with us that he would need a clean-cut image to work in an environment peopled with parents and children.

Whenever I dropped him off at work, he always insisted that I get back in the car once I'd taken his wheelchair out of the car trunk and leave him alone to negotiate the ramp that had been installed for him. In case anyone was watching, he didn't want them to think that he couldn't do such things without help from his mom. So I'd drop him off; then I'd sit in the car to watch and wait as he struggled slowly up the ramp in his manually operated wheelchair. Once he'd reached the top of the ramp, he couldn't enter the building until he'd wrestled to open a very large and heavy door. Yet at moments like these, I was fiercely proud of his determination to do these difficult things independent of me.

Mike loved working at the Y, but like the Little League coaching that he'd also loved, it came to an abrupt end several months after he started work. He called me one evening and said not to bother picking him up after work, that one of his friends would be coming after him. He gave no indication that anything was wrong, but he avoided us by staying out most of the night and by sleeping very late the next morning. When finally I decided I'd better wake him up so he could get ready for work, he grumbled sleepily, "I don't work there anymore," and turned over and went back to sleep.

What now? I wondered as I closed his bedroom door and slumped onto a kitchen chair to consider this unexpected development.

When he came out of his room much later, he told us that the kindly woman who was executive director at the Y had called him into her office and told him that she was very sorry but that there had been objections to his being at the front desk and that it had been decided by board members that he could continue on the job only if he agreed to work in the back room.

"Who complained? And why?" I asked angrily.

He shrugged. "Who cares who and why? What matters is that they think I'm a freak who has to be hidden away in a back room out of sight of the children."

"That can't be it, Mike. Maybe someone said something about your partying reputation . . ."

"Maybe so," he admitted. "But no matter what, I won't be shut away in a back room. So I guess I'm out of a job."

I asked him if he wanted me to intervene with the executive director, whom I'd come to know and admire, but he said it was over and done with and to leave it alone. I wanted desperately to know if what he had told me was true, but I respected his wishes and didn't pursue finding out why he had left his Y job even though it bothered me a great deal not to.

After that, he let his hair and beard grow back and left home to live in a run-down motel where unemployed transients lived. When we objected to his moving there, he reacted to our protests with "Why shouldn't I? I'm a reject the same as everyone else living there! Besides, that's all I can afford."

I have to confess that though it was difficult, I tried to put Mike out of my mind for a while after that. Our other son, Dick, was still at home, and Cindy would be coming home to spend part of her summer break from college, and I wanted to enjoy our time with them without having Mike's ever-constant problems hanging over our heads.

Besides, there was some pleasant OIF work to be done. I was in my second year as OIF president and had scheduled a July board meeting in Chicago that required my attention. I hoped that meeting in person at the site where OIF had come to life would give our new directors a positive boost and recharge the veterans. At the invitation of Drs. Millar and Sofield, the Medical Advisory Board agreed to attend, to review, and to make recommendations on grant applications, an activity that had previously been done by mail. It promised to be quite a meeting, and it was. A record-breaking number of grants were approved, and some very important strategic planning took place. Driving home late that sultry Sunday evening after the meeting, I felt more relaxed about the future of OIF than I had in a long time. The caliber of expertise demonstrated by our medical advisors and directors had been so impressive.

I was still on cloud nine when we arrived home around midnight and found young Dick still up and waiting for us. Usually laid-back, he seemed overly anxious. "Thank God, you're finally home," he said. "I've been so worried!"

His unusual concern surprised me. "Why were you worried? We've driven to Chicago and back more times than I can count. It never worried you before."

Smiling wanly, he hedged. "I don't know. I tried going to bed, but I couldn't sleep. So I decided to wait up for you."

I kidded him. "Now you know what we go through when you're out past your curfew."

"Yeah, I sure do," he sighed.

"Well, we're home safe and sound now, so you can go to bed," his father told him. "That's where I'm going. I'm bushed!"

Still seeming concerned, our youngest son turned to me. "Mom, I . . ."

Sensing that he had something else to say, I asked, "What is it?"

He shrugged. "How was your meeting?"

"Excellent! One of the best so far!" I exclaimed.

Again, he repeated, "Mom . . ." then stopped.

"Dick, what is it?" I begged.

He gave another small shrug. "Never mind. Good night, Mom!" he said and took the steps two at a time in his haste to get upstairs.

I had taken off from work the next morning and was lazily sitting at the kitchen table having a second cup of coffee while listening to a program on the local radio station that gave the kind of information small towns are noted for—hospital admittances, deaths, births, traffic violations, and other arrests—when I thought I heard Mike's name. Jumping from my chair, I turned up the volume in time to hear the announcer say that Mike had been arrested for possession of marijuana at the motel where he lived.

Sinking back into my chair, I realized that this was probably what Dick had known but hadn't been able to tell us the previous night; and I wept, not for Mike this time, but for the rest of us who would have to endure a new round of undeserved and unwanted public scrutiny. "So, God," I murmured bitterly as I wept, "is this your answer to my prayers?"

When he came home from work, Dick looked grim, so I knew right away that he knew. "I suppose I should go find out where he is and bail him out," he said wearily.

I didn't want any part of it, but for my husband's sake, I asked, "Do you want me to go with you?"

He hesitated only briefly. "No, you stay here. I'll handle it," he gently said.

When he came back several hours later, he told me, "I found him at the jail and got him a lawyer. I wanted to bring him home, but he refused and had me take him back to that stinking motel."

"Is he okay?"

"Not really. You should have seen him. What a sight. I don't think he had showered or shaved for a week or more. I talked to Don [his cousin who was sheriff at the time], and he advised me to get him out of that motel before he gets in deeper, but I don't know how we're going to do that. He sure wouldn't come home with me."

Cindy arrived later that week, and when she was told what had happened, she volunteered to go to the motel to bring Mike home.

"I'm going with you," I told her, and she agreed to let me accompany her.

At the motel, we pounded on the door of his room but got no answer. The woman in the motel office assured us that Mike was in his room and, knowing who we were, offered to unlock the door when she heard why we were there.

All the drapes in the room were drawn, making it so dark it was hard to see as we walked through the door, leaving the bright sunlight behind. Out of the darkness rose a stench of stale pizza and cigarette smoke. On the rumpled bed, something moved under a sheet. Then came an exclamation of surprise as Cindy drew open the drapes to let some light in. Gently, she pulled the sheet off the lump on the bed and said, "Mike, it's Cindy . . . and Mom."

Looking dazed and disheveled, he sat up and demanded, "How did you get in here?"

"We knocked, and when you didn't answer, we got worried," Cindy said as she planted a kiss on his cheek. "So we asked the lady in the office to open the door for us. I wanted to see you. I hope you don't mind."

Smiling wanly, he said, "Naw, it's okay."

Wasting no time, Cindy said, "Mom and I are here to bring you home."

"No way!" he exploded. "My rent is paid up here, and this is where I'm staying!"

Noticing that he had slept in his clothes, I said, "Just slide into your wheelchair and let's go."

He was adamant. "I am not leaving! All my stuff is here."

"I'm home for only a few days, come spend them with me," Cindy pleaded. "If you decide to stay, we'll come back and get your stuff. If not, I'll bring you back. I promise."

Mike was a mess like Dick had said, so when he finally, but still reluctantly, agreed to come home with us, Cindy and I wheeled him into the drive-in shower Dick had constructed for him in our attached garage before we let him enter the house. After his shower, we got the scissors out and cut his long shaggy hair amid a tirade of protests, then gave him clean clothes to wear. Maybe, unconsciously, we hoped that this cleansing would reveal the old Mike whom we had known and loved for so long. But of course, deep down, we knew that it would take more than a good scrubbing to accomplish that.

Chapter Twenty-Four

When Cindy returned to college after the weekend, Mike stayed. During their many conversations those two days, Cindy had apparently convinced him to go after what he really wanted—his independence. He was going to talk to his rehab counselor, he said, about taking driving lessons, getting his license, and eventually acquiring a car with hand controls. Happy about the sudden reversal, Dick promised that he would help him get a car and would make whatever modifications were needed so he could drive it.

"Thanks anyway, Dad," he said with an appreciative smile. "But I plan to finance it with a bank loan, and rehab will pay to have the hand controls installed. It's all set. But you can help me figure out how to get in the car and then haul my wheelchair in after myself so I can drive alone, okay?"

Several weeks later, he was taking driving lessons, and he told us that after talking to his rehab counselor, he had agreed to go back to college in Lima to pick up where he'd left off.

"How are you going to get back and forth?" I asked. "You still don't have a driver's license or car."

"My counselor says he can arrange for me to stay at a group home in Lima temporarily until I have wheels and can find an apartment there," he said.

Surprised that he would agree to that kind of arrangement, I said, "Group homes have rules and curfews, are you sure you can handle that?"

He grinned. "No more parties. Right?"

"Right!"

Confidentially, he added, "I won't be there long. But it's part of the deal I had to make to be able to take driving lessons and get a car. No college and no group home mean no driving lessons and no car. It's that simple."

"So the only reason you're going back to college is to get a car?" I asked, unable to hide my disappointment.

He paused, then looked away. "I admit it," he confessed. "Getting a car was the main reason I agreed to go back to school. But maybe I'll get lucky and get something out of my courses this time."

I wanted to scold him and hug him all at the same time. But I didn't do either one. For years, he'd been dealing to get what he wanted, and most of the time, his deals had brought him nothing but trouble. Yet he was still hopeful that some good would come from this latest one.

"So what kind of place is this group home?" I asked.

Again, he shifted his eyes. "It's a temporary place," he repeated, "where state rehab clients go to live until they can find other arrangements. My counselor promised to help me find an apartment so I won't have to be there long."

An alarm went off somewhere in the recesses of my mind. "What is it, a halfway house?"

"Sort of."

"What do you mean sort of?"

"A few parolees live there, I guess, and others with mental or emotional problems, but most are people like me, going to school and waiting for better housing to become available."

Worried by the apparent notoriety of some of the residents, I said, "Let's go look at the place before you move in, make sure it's accessible and safe."

"Oh, Mom," he sighed, "I've already agreed to live there, and I did check it out. It'll be okay until I can find another place. You can see it for yourself when you and Dad help me take my stuff over. You will take me over, won't you?"

"Sure," I replied, but I still wasn't convinced that this "group home," or whatever it was, was the place for him.

"Mom, it's really not that bad," he said reassuringly. "It's a palace compared to some of the dumps I've lived in, and they serve three meals a day!"

The group home was an old house located in a middle-class neighborhood, and on the fall afternoon that we took Mike to live there, it seemed unusually quiet for a group home. When I casually remarked about it, the house parent told us that the residents went out to lunch, then to a movie, or the mall, or some other such activity every Sunday.

Almost too brightly, as if to convince himself as well as us, Mike said, "See, I won't be stuck here with nothing to do or nowhere to go."

Though the furniture in the bedroom he was assigned to seemed somewhat abused, the room and beds appeared clean. The house parent who showed us around told Mike that it would be his responsibility to make his bed and keep his clothes picked up and that he would have to participate in the scheduled house meetings and take his turn helping in the kitchen. "And of course, you already know that we won't be responsible for the loss or theft of any valuables," he concluded.

Mike wouldn't even consider sending his most valuable possession, a small color TV he was buying on an installment plan, back home with us. Nor did we urge him to, knowing that the Baseball World Series were in progress and that the football season too had already begun.

On the way home, I had an uneasy feeling about having abandoned him there. It was a feeling similar to the one I'd often experienced when leaving him at the hospital for lengthy bouts of surgery. I knew he'd be hurting, living under so many restraints, yet I was hopeful about the outcome. Mike was right, I told myself, when he said that he had lived in worst places. So I pushed my ambivalence aside, decided that structured living would be good for him, and tried to focus on his long-range plans with optimism.

The day a large silver gray Chrysler Cordoba pulled into our driveway and Mike emerged from it the triumphant owner, I firmly believed that it justified the move to the group home. I hadn't seen him look this proud and happy since that long ago day when, at age four, he had walked unaided down the long corridor at Shriners Hospital.

"It's so big!" I exclaimed. "How are you ever going to be able to control such a big car? Besides, you don't even know if you're going to get your license yet!"

"I'll get it soon," he said confidently. "Until then, some of my friends have agreed to drive me around."

For the first time since the car had pulled into the driveway, I peered in at the stranger sitting behind the wheel. "Hi!" I cordially greeted him. "So you've volunteered to drive this big bucket of bolts?"

With a cocky grin, the driver replied, "I don't mind, as long as he pays me."

My jaw dropped. Mike had himself a car *and* a paid chauffeur! The look on my face must have exposed what I was thinking. Laughing, Mike quickly explained, "Mom, he's just one of the guys from the group home. I needed someone to drive me over here, so I gave him a couple of bucks. No big deal, okay?" Then turning to his father, he asked, "So what do you think, Dad?"

"It's a big car. A smaller make would have been a lot easier for you to handle," Dick said cautiously.

"You want to take a look under the hood?" Mike prodded. "Check the tires, that kind of thing?"

"We should have done all of that *before* you bought it," Dick reprimanded as he lifted the hood and began checking things out. He tinkered around the motor, then appearing satisfied, put the hood back in place. "The motor looks good, and everything seems to be working fine," he said. "Tires look almost new, so they should last a while. Now what about the inside? How are we going to fix it so you can get yourself in and out and sit high enough to see out the windows?"

The stranger got out of the car to allow them to inspect the interior, but I hardly gave him a glance, I was too busy trying to figure out why Mike had chosen this big silver gray machine as his first car. Did the size give him an elusion of power and strength, or did he imagine it to be the silver chariot that would finally transport him to all the faraway places he had dreamed about?

Later, as we stood in the driveway and watched the car disappear around the corner, Dick marveled, "I never thought I'd see the day when Mike would have his own car."

"Especially not a silver chariot with a chauffeur," I laughed.

Dick smiled broadly. "It looks more like an army tank to me."

Army tank or chariot, owning a car proved to be a positive thing for Mike. With it as incentive, he quickly finished his driving course, obtained his license, got rehab to install the hand controls, and worked with his father on a plan for a lift to help him load and unload his wheelchair into the car unassisted.

Every time the silver gray tank, as we fondly called the car, appeared in our driveway, I would be amazed all over again by Mike's newfound independence. Yet I also was fearfully aware that such a powerful vehicle could be dangerous, so I was always relieved when he came accompanied by someone. Though a few of his old friends sometimes came with him, most of the people he now brought to our house were other residents of the group home. Of the two that accompanied him most often, one was dark and sullen, and rarely spoke. I surmised that his disability was either mental or emotional, and I was nervous about Mike spending any time at all with him. The other was a small-statured boy with long light brown hair named Terry, who appeared to be barely out of his teens and who definitely had a sunnier disposition. Mike confided to me that he had befriended Terry, who had been abandoned by his family and raised in abusive foster homes, and was trying to help him rebuild his self-esteem. When I good-naturedly teased him about turning into a do-gooder, he teased back, "Yeah, just like my mom!"

Knowing that Mike was trying to help him, we didn't mind having Terry come into our home. Sometimes the two of them would breeze in and out for a quick visit; other times, they stayed for lunch. Once, when Mike had brought his car over for his father to make minor repairs, I drove the two of them back to Lima. It was a pleasantly satisfying trip with a lot of easy banter and jokes about the happenings at the group home.

It wasn't until Mike spent time alone with us during the holidays that he began to drop hints and make vague references about some of the not-so-funny incidents that were occurring at the group home and about the weird behavior of some of the residents. Some of his things had been stolen, so he had bought locks and keys to protect his other belongings, and he was keeping his money tucked safely under his pillow when he slept at night. Someone had put sand in the gas tank of his car as a prank, and getting it cleaned out had been costly. Then one day, he'd asked one of the residents if he wanted to go riding around with him and had ended up several hundred miles away in Kentucky.

"Kentucky! How on earth did you end up in Kentucky?" I cried.

"He just wanted to go there, that's all. No big deal. I shouldn't have told you. Now you'll worry."

What Mike didn't tell me until much later was that the man he had driven to Kentucky was an ex-convict intent on visiting his family after having served a prison term for manslaughter.

When the New Year began, Mike started it with a long list of resolutions. He had a feeling, he said, that this was going to be his year. Determined to turn his life around, he broke off relationships he thought were detrimental and started to work at rekindling those he valued. With a gleam in his eyes, he advised everyone that he was going to lose weight and find himself a girlfriend. Now and again, when we asked how the girlfriend search was going, he glumly replied that he had asked several for a date and had been turned down flat. After seeing the movie *Saturday Night Fever*, he wondered what it would be like to have girls falling all over him the way they did over John Travolta; but even in his wildest dreams, he said he couldn't imagine anything that wonderful ever happening to him. But still he kept trying. Once he was reinstated in college, he began searching in earnest for a part-time job and an apartment of his own.

When he revealed that he was not only sleeping with his money, but also with a knife under his pillow for protection, we were appalled and scared, and we urged him to check out of there. "I'm talking to my rehab counselor about it. He knows the situation, and he's spending a lot of time trying to find me an accessible apartment in Lima so I won't have to commute back and forth. Coming back home won't solve anything," he finished with a sad smile, yet I sensed that the offer was tempting to him.

Without telling Mike, I phoned his rehab counselor to find out if the horrific conditions he described truly existed. Reluctantly, he replied that yes, there were some unsavory characters living there, and that Mike shouldn't really be there, but that there was nothing else available at the moment. He assured me, however, that he was working very hard to help him find a nice, respectable place to live and that he thought he had located one that would soon be available. When I suggested that he talk Mike into coming home until the apartment was ready, he informed me that they had discussed that possibility but that Mike had told him that moving back home wasn't part of his plan to become totally self-sufficient, so he had opted to stay put until the apartment was his. Mike was determined to be his own man, his counselor said, to have his own place and live his own life, and that his job as Mike's counselor was to help him achieve those goals. "However," he finished kindly, "it's good to know that he has a place to go to in an emergency."

The next time I saw Mike, I suggested that he ask God to help him find a job and an apartment. Scoffing loudly, he said, "When has praying ever helped me?"

"Try again," I insisted. "Maybe, this time God will hear . . ."

"And say no," he said, flatly finishing my sentence.

Sometime later, Mike's rehab counselor phoned to say that they were running out of time, that Mike would have to leave the group home because state inspectors were coming. When I asked why he would have to leave because of the inspectors' visit, he sheepishly acknowledged that the home was a mental health facility and that Mike should not have been placed there in the first place since his disability was physical and not mental. He asked if the offer to have Mike come back home to live was still good, and of course, I said yes, that we would come after him right away. "Not yet," he said. He had phoned to ascertain whether the offer was still in effect in case Mike had nowhere else to go, but first, he wanted to check up on the availability of the apartment he had applied for and to find out whether a promising job interview Mike had recently had with the IRS might result in a job offer.

Ecstatic, Mike phoned several days later to tell us that he had gotten the IRS job and that the apartment would be his on April 1. "Mom, it's all coming together finally," he said happily.

Paraphrasing the words of Martin Luther King, Jr., I joked, "Free at last! Thank God Almighty you're free at last!"

I heard the sound of a chuckle over the telephone wire. "You sound happy," he said. "Are you?"

"Yes, I'm very happy for you Mike *and* very relieved that you're getting out of that group home."

"So am I," he sighed, and this time, I heard great relief in his voice.

By April 1, Mike was installed in his new apartment. The Friday of that week was the beginning of the Easter weekend, and Mike came to spend it with us. "Mom," he said when we had a quiet moment alone, "I wanted to tell you something, but I didn't want to do it when everyone else was here. But I can't think of a better time than this Easter weekend to tell you . . ." He hesitated, seemed shy when he asked, "You're not gonna laugh, are you?"

I sensed that he had something difficult to say. "No, I won't laugh. I promise."

Encouraged, he asked, "Remember when you suggested that I pray for God's help to find an apartment and a job?"

"I remember."

"Well, I did, and right away, my apartment became available, and I got a job!" he exclaimed.

I smiled. "You, the agnostic, prayed?"

"Yup, I did," he acknowledged. "And things have been going great ever since. My college courses are going well. I now have a neat apartment. I drive my own car, and I even have a job." Again, shyly, he added, "If you don't mind, I'd like to go to church with you and Dad on Easter Sunday."

"Mike, that would be wonderful," I said and planted a grateful kiss on him.

"Don't get mushy with me," he said, but I could tell that he was just as pleased with the turn of events as I was.

The following Sunday, April 13, was Mike's twenty-fourth birthday, and he had invited us to come see his new apartment. So armed with housewarming and birthday gifts and a birthday cake, we drove to Lima, accompanied by Cathy and her three children. Jennifer, Emily, and Ryan loved their Uncle Mike, and they couldn't wait to get there for his birthday party. When Mike greeted us at the door of his second-floor apartment, he was thrilled to see them too, and he joked with them and tried to guess what was in the gaily wrapped presents we had brought for him.

While the children clamored to get the party going, Mike gave us a quick tour of his apartment. Later, after the presents had been opened and everyone was satisfyingly full of cake and ice cream, he proudly showed us the personal touches he had added.

Among them was a refrigerator filled with healthy, wholesome food; a sunny windowsill graced with two small flowering plants; and a framed art print, on loan from the local library, hanging on the pale yellow living room wall. When he saw the painting by one of the old masters, Dick winked at me and raised his eyebrows at the drastic change in Mike's taste in wall hangings. But I could tell that he was pleased as I was to see the effort Mike was putting into changing his lifestyle.

As we prepared to leave, we cautioned him not to get stuck in the pull-down bed that folded back out of sight into the wall when not in use. With good humor, he replied that we shouldn't worry, that he was planning to take his phone to bed with him so he could call for help in case the unthinkable did happen. Hugging and kissing him one more time, we finally said good-bye.

During the drive home, I uttered a silent prayer of thanksgiving. "Thank you, Lord, for answering Mike's prayers and for finally allowing him the freedom to live his own life."

Having said that, I let myself sink into a pleasant mix of peace and contentment because our job raising Mike had come to such a satisfying conclusion. It was so much easier to let go now that Mike had placed himself safely back into God's hands.

Epilogue

Only one month later, on May 14, 1980, while Dick and I were in Las Cruces, New Mexico, attending Cindy's college graduation, Mike was fatally beaten by Terry Polm, one of the residents of the group home where he had briefly resided. This young man, whom we had welcomed into our home, killed Mike in a premeditated assault to rob him of a small sum of money and a newly purchased stereo.

And so it was with breaking hearts that we laid Mike to rest on a beautiful, sun-drenched morning in May, ending twenty-four self-revealing, painful, yet hopeful years of life with Mike and osteogenesis imperfecta. Words are not adequate to express the anger and agony that we felt. Mixed with the tears and the incredible grief were the recriminations and the incessant questions.

Why Mike? Why now after he'd had such a meager taste of independence? Was it our fault for letting him go? What if we had objected more strenuously against his living in the group home, especially after he had told us about his fears of living there? What if we had been more vocal about his coming back home while he waited for an apartment to become available? The list of whys and what-ifs was long, varied, and—in the end—futile. For no matter how much we wondered about the possible outcomes of the choices not made, nothing could ever change what had happened.

There were many who advised me to leave the foundation work behind, suggesting that with Mike gone, I had no further need to be involved. Only my family and my closest friends knew what the work meant to me. Having been the messengers of hope had given meaning to our lives. Being able to tell other families like us that, finally, there was something *we* could do, was important and gratifying. So the decision was made to go on.

Routinely working every day to help others in need kept me from caving in when we had to relive the nightmarish details of Mike's death during the October trial of Terry Polm. After three grueling days of devastating testimony, Polm was convicted of aggravated murder and sentenced to life imprisonment.

To say that we felt justice had been done or that closure had been achieved would be claiming a resolution that we would not feel for many years. So to find the healing that I so desperately needed, I buried myself in the work of the OI Foundation. During the lonely, sometimes endless, days that followed, it was Dick, our children, my faith in God, and my OIF family that lifted me up and urged me to continue when I thought I could not.

To honor Mike's memory and to continue the research work we had helped to initiate, the board of directors voted, in 1981, to establish the Mike Geisman Memorial Fellowship Fund to encourage young researchers, working under the direction of senior scientists, to study the many complexities of osteogenesis imperfecta.

Knowing that Mike's life journey had not always been exemplary, I hesitated to accept the honor at first. Yet deep in my heart, I knew from my *Redbook* experiences that admitting mistakes and acknowledging failures can sometimes be powerful building tools. Even though Mike was gone, many others could benefit by letting him live on in this way. So we agreed to allow his name to be used to represent all individuals who live with the many challenges of osteogenesis imperfecta.

I never intended to continue working for the OI Foundation for as long as I did. But whenever I thought of resigning, something or someone always drew me back in. For instance, in 1982, Nelda Rohm, who was president of the board at the time, persuaded me to work with her to organize a national conference for teens and adults with OI. A growing number of them had been clamoring for an opportunity to get together to talk about living independently, going to college, having a career, finding a job, dating, and—yes—marriage. Even though I knew that being around young people who, like Mike, dreamed of an independent life of their own would be extremely difficult, I reluctantly agreed to do it.

Over fifty teens and young adults with OI, some accompanied by their parents, came to that first national conference in Little Rock, Arkansas. For some of them, it was their first time away from home; and when the conference ended three days later, they didn't want to leave until we promised to have another conference the following year. Meeting and talking with others who had OI had changed their lives, they said. New friendships had been forged. They had been given new hope and a limitless amount of possibilities. So we promised to do it again, and we did. Encouraged by the success of the first two conferences, it was decided to make the next meetings all inclusive by opening them up to entire families, medical professionals, and friends and to hold the meetings biannually instead of yearly. These proved to be even more popular. The Washington, D.C., conference held in 2008 was the largest so far with over seven hundred in attendance!

In the fall of 1982, when Dick and I moved from Ohio to New Hampshire, I was asked to move the OIF office with me and continue working in the dual position of executive director and *Breakthrough* editor until replacements could be found. Had I known that it would take four more years, I doubt that I would have agreed. At the time, I had begun to write this book, and I wanted to return to school to take creative writing and public speaking courses, which I eventually did.

Though I wanted to make a clean break from OIF when I again offered up my resignation in 1986, the members of the board refused it and instead reinstated me as a member of the board. I was now the only remaining founding member actively involved in the development of the OI Foundation. Dick, my most ardent cheerleader, agreed with them that I should stay on. Reluctantly, I accepted their decision even though I believed that it was time for new people to take over.

A year later, at a meeting in Tampa, where the president of OIF, my friend and colleague Rosalind James of New York, had spearheaded the establishment of new headquarters for OIF, the board members again countered my postponed resignation by unanimously voting to grant me lifetime membership on the board. It would be a voting position, they said, with no other demands on my time. It was an offer I couldn't refuse. So I accepted and continued writing my book.

Though I intended my role to be a passive one, it turned out to be anything but that. It soon became apparent that I still had some battles to fight. At each turn in the road, Dick and my many loyal foundation friends kept pushing and urging me to fight for what we believed in.

When the new leadership of OIF decided to rename the foundation with a generic "brittle bone" name, I led the charge to keep the osteogenesis imperfecta label. We won, but my popularity with the leadership went into a very sharp decline.

When something seemed contrary to the OIF mission or bylaws, I spoke up on behalf of my fellow founding members who could no longer speak for themselves. I won some and lost some, made new allies and some adversaries in the process.

I heard about grumblings among the ranks. I was keeping the foundation from making progress by clinging to the old ways. I was against rebranding OIF. Behind the scenes, some were saying that it was time for the "old lady" to go. A close foundation colleague used to kid me with the reminder that they were trying to "throw Mama from the train," the title of a popular movie at the time.

When the board of directors decided to move the national office to the Washington DC area and hire another executive director, it seemed the perfect time for me to get off the train. I should have, but I didn't. Things were going so well under the direction of Joe Antolini, Sid Simmons, Jean-Paul Richard, and others. So much was being accomplished, and I wanted to finally be able to sit back and enjoy being part of history in the making. Our hard work was finally paying off. The publications, the Web site, the national conferences, and the Mike Geisman Memorial Fellowship Fund were making a huge difference in the lives of OI families. It was all so exhilarating and exciting to watch. Why should I get off now? Especially when OIF was finally on the right track and headed in the right direction?

By then, I knew without doubt that the child who had once been perceived a burden, had instead been a bearer of gifts for us and for all who are affected with osteogenesis imperfecta. I knew that because Mike and the children of the other founding families had lived, a successful support network was in place for those who needed it. Medical information about OI was readily available in *Breakthrough*, the brochures and other literature, most of which were easily accessible on the internet. Because Mike had died, there was a research fund, established in his memory, that was bringing with it the hope that someday a cure would be found.

Of more importance to our family, however, were the valuable things that we had learned while Mike was with us. Had it not been for him, I doubted that we would have discovered what real commitment to a cause and true compassion for those who suffer really meant. And, most likely, we would never have acquired the ability to see and appreciate the uniqueness of individuals, regardless of their physical characteristics. Above all else, living with Mike had certainly taught us how to love unconditionally and had given us the good sense of knowing when to hold on and when to let go. For all these reasons, I once again decided to stay with OIF because I wanted to share with others what I had learned along the way.

In 1999, Dick and I retired to Florida, and I finished my book and got an agent who was very enthusiastic about getting it published. New York publishers liked it but felt it should be aimed at a "special" readership within the OI and other disability communities. So we began submitting it to smaller publishers, who also liked it but suggested that self-publishing might be the best way to go. Somewhat dispirited by the rejections, I put the manuscript in our safe-deposit box and told myself that maybe I would self-publish it "someday."

During that time, Dick constantly urged me to get it out and do something with it. "Send it out again," he'd nag. "Your story needs to be told!" But I held off. I wasn't sure I wanted to relive it all over again. I wanted to be free to enjoy our well-earned retirement years in the sunshine.

The decision to keep it locked away was made for me when Dick was diagnosed with pulmonary fibrosis, a rare and incurable lung disease, and given only a few short years to live. Though I was still on the board of directors at the time, it had become increasingly apparent that I was no longer needed. So I resigned my mostly honorary position and made Dick's remaining years my loving priority.

They were difficult, yet peaceful years, filled with many quiet days spent counting our blessings and talking about our life choices and the lessons we had learned from them. We marveled at how lucky we had been to have found each other and how fortunate that our whirlwind courtship had blossomed and matured into a very special partnership that had lasted over fifty-five years and produced four beautiful children and twelve very special grandchildren. During these talks, we often spoke of Mike, smiling now as we recounted some of the things he had done, how comical yet seriously determined he had been, and yes, we also sadly remembered how foolish and dangerous some of his choices and decisions had been.

We now spoke of him and the OI Foundation as gifts—gifts that would never die, but would keep on giving for years to come. We marveled at the amazing research being funded by the Mike Geisman Memorial Fellowship Fund, the linked clinics where patients and their families could get the medical treatments they needed, the hugely popular and successful conferences, the innovative fund-raisers, and the astonishing number of volunteers who were continuing the work that we had so idealistically undertaken years ago. Most of our talks ended with Dick reminding me to take "our book" out of mothballs, update it, and send it out again. My answer was always "Maybe. Someday."

When he died peacefully at home on September 30, 2008, with our daughter Cathy and I by his side, I knew that "someday" was near. It was now or never. And so it is for him that I publish this book, for without him, Mike, our other children, Cathy, Cindy, and Rick, this journey would not have been undertaken or this story told.

I also dedicate it to my cofounders, fellow directors and officers, and the many others who, throughout the years, stepped in and kept things going when we thought all was lost. I especially want to remember those who gave so much but are no longer here to witness the continuing success of the OI Foundation. After all, it is their story too.

Author's Note

The research initiative discussed in this story did not prove to be an effective long term treatment or cure for osteogenesis imperfecta. However, it was Dr. Edward Millar's and Dr.Clive Solomons's willingness to help a despairing group of parents that opened up the laboratories of other researchers interested in the study of OI. For information about ongoing OI research, other programs and services, or to become a volunteer for OIF, Inc., please go to www.oif.org.